HOW WE CAN LIVE WITH ARTHRITIS

The Easy Guide To Managing Symptoms Better

BY
A.D. HUTCHINSON

Table of Contents

INTRODUCTION

Arthritis affects people of all ages, from children to the elderly. It is not a single sickness but rather a broad range of ailments, each with its traits and effects. As one of the main causes of disability worldwide, arthritis is a serious health burden, with millions of people dealing with its effects on a daily basis.

Arthritis has a centuries-long history, with evidence found in ancient Egyptian mummies and classical civilization books. However, in the nineteenth and twentieth centuries, medical knowledge of arthritis began to progress drastically. Diagnostic breakthroughs such as X-rays and blood testing transformed the diagnosis and treatment of various types of arthritis.

In 1982, Alan Douglas Hutchinson from London, England, was diagnosed with Rheumatoid Arthritis in his index finger on his right hand. It became swollen and sometimes very blistered. In a matter of months, it spread to all his fingers on both hands, then to all his toes, including his big toes. Over the years, it spread to every joint in his body, including his elbows, knees, neck, ankles, and jaws. He could not walk for five years; he used to creep like a child in and around the house for over five years. Alan is still able to move around without assistance, and he is in less pain now than he was when it all began forty years ago. He does not smoke, drink alcohol, or add sugar to his tea or coffee. He works out frequently and consumes a lot of fruits, vegetables, and nuts. He eats less fried foods and more grilled or steamed foods.

Over the past 40 years, he has tried numerous alternative medicines and treatments, from gold injections to steroids. He would do as much movement and activities as possible rather than sitting down for a long period. Some people suffer from damaging joints with deformities caused by Rheumatoid and Psoriatic arthritis, but others don't suffer from any deformity whatsoever. Although it's been over 40 years since Alan was diagnosed with arthritis, he never walks with any walking aids, such as a walking stick or crutch stick. Many people are wheelchair users because of arthritis; some are unable to move without support. Arthritis is much worse in the summer, with mild pains in winter.

Even though arthritis is still incurable, recent developments in treatment have significantly improved patient outcomes. Early diagnosis and intervention are critical for effective illness management, particularly for inflammatory forms of arthritis such as rheumatoid arthritis. Numerous therapies, including physical therapy, medication, and lifestyle modifications, can help patients feel better and lessen symptoms.

In addition to medical interventions, arthritis support groups can help people cope with the problems of the condition. These groups offer essential information, emotional support, and practical help to persons suffering from arthritis. In the United Kingdom, two notable organisations, Arthritis Action UK and Versus Arthritis UK, stand out for their dedication to helping arthritis patients.

Despite these developments, having arthritis still comes with a lot of difficulties. The erratic nature of the symptoms, which can change drastically on a daily basis, can cause disruptions to daily schedules and negatively affect general well-being and well-being. Furthermore, because many forms of arthritis are chronic, long-term management measures are necessary, which puts a heavy load on both patients and healthcare systems.

This guide's admirable goal is to lend a supportive hand to people who have arthritis by offering advice and different coping mechanisms for the pain and discomfort that this illness often causes. Through a proper understanding of the subtleties of arthritis and adopting various coping strategies, individuals with the condition can set out on a path to better health and a higher standard of living.

CHAPTER 1:
WHAT IS ARTHRITIS?
Understanding the Term Arthritis

Arthritis is a medical disorder that causes acute or chronic inflammation in one or more joints.

In essence, "arthritis" is only a slang term for joint pain or sickness. There are over 100 different types of arthritis and related disorders. Arthritis is the biggest cause of disability worldwide and affects people of all ages, genders, and races. The precise number of arthritis patients is unknown since many people wait until their symptoms deteriorate before seeking treatment.

Every May, the United States observes National Arthritis Awareness Month to increase public awareness of the condition and the enormous toll it takes on millions of lives. The campaign has a strong emphasis on informing the public about the vital roles that early diagnosis, treatment, and lifestyle modifications have in the efficient management of conditions.

Common symptoms of joint arthritis include swelling, pain, stiffness, and restricted range of motion. There are three gradations of symptoms: mild, moderate, and severe. They can also get worse over time or stay constant for years. Walking and climbing stairs can be challenging when arthritis flares up to a degree that is too intense for regular duties. In addition, arthritis may result in long-term abnormalities of the joints; some are evident (e.g., finger joints that are knobby), while others need to be seen using an X-ray. Other organs like the heart, eyes, lungs, kidneys, and skin can also be impacted by certain types of arthritis.

While arthritis has no known cure, there are many treatments that can help control symptoms and improve overall quality of life. In order to empower you on your path to greater wellbeing, this chapter will explore essential insights. Now, let's get started on this educational journey!

The Prevalence and Impact of Arthritis

Arthritis includes over 100 conditions that affect the joints and surrounding tissues. It is a primary source of chronic pain, disability, and limitations on one's activities. It is also linked to the prescription of opioids, which significantly raises the expense of healthcare.

The word "arthritis" often refers to inflammation of one or more joints, resulting in pain, stiffness, edoema, and decreased range of motion. The four most common kinds of arthritis are osteoarthritis, rheumatoid arthritis, psoriatic arthritis and gout. As an inflammatory disorder, RA produces inflammation of the joints as the body's immune system attacks its tissues. In contrast, OA mostly affects the cartilage within the joints, causing it to break down over time. Some people with gout may also have psoriasis, an inflammatory skin disorder brought on by uric acid crystal buildup in the joints.

People of any age, gender, or race can be affected by arthritis, although it is more common in older people. Over 54 million Americans suffer from arthritis, making it a common chronic ailment, according to the Centres for Disease Control and Prevention (CDC). Around 350 million people worldwide suffer from osteoarthritis, which is the most common type of arthritis.

Beyond just causing physical pain, arthritis has a substantial negative influence on people's quality of life, productivity, and socioeconomic standing. Pain and stiffness associated with chronic arthritis can limit mobility, making it challenging to do everyday tasks, work, and participate in social and recreational activities. Moreover, arthritis is among the world's leading causes of disability, increasing the demand for medical services, decreasing productivity, and increasing absenteeism.

Additionally, arthritis places a significant financial strain on society at large and healthcare institutions. Medical expenses related to arthritis can be classified as direct or indirect. Direct expenditures include hospital stays, doctor visits, drugs, and surgery; indirect costs include disability payments, missed work, and caregiving responsibilities.

The overall burden of arthritis is further increased by the tight association between arthritis and mental health conditions, including anxiety and depression. The physical restrictions brought on by arthritis and persistent pain can cause social isolation, frustration, and powerlessness, all of which can negatively affect one's mental health and general quality of life. Further impairing their capacity to operate at their best are the possibility of weariness, cognitive impairment, and sleep difficulties in those with arthritis.

Arthritis continues to be a major public health concern with many unmet requirements despite advancements in medical therapy and management techniques. In order to improve outcomes and lower the worldwide burden of arthritis, research endeavours focused on clarifying the pathophysiology of various arthritic disorders, finding new therapeutic targets, and creating individualised treatment approaches are essential.

Arthritis is a major global public health concern due to its high prevalence, severe impact on productivity and quality of life, and large financial cost. For people with arthritis, symptom relief, maintaining joint function, and general wellbeing are contingent upon the implementation of effective management techniques that include early diagnosis, multimodal therapy approaches, and holistic care.

Causes and Risk Factors for Developing Arthritis

As mentioned above, there are over a hundred different types of arthritis, each with unique causes and risk factors. Therefore, determining the cause of arthritis can be difficult since multiple overlapping factors typically contribute to its development. Infections, traumas, autoimmune disorders, and wear and tear caused by aging and lifestyle choices are all possible causes of arthritis. Let's take a look at this one after the other.

Common Causes

Although other causes and risk factors are associated with each of the main types of arthritis, these are the most frequently observed.

- ♦ Age Factor

The natural aging process, which causes changes in the structure and function of joints, increases the risk of arthritis. As we age, the cartilage, which cushions the ends of bones in joints, gradually thins and loses its strength. People with this deterioration are more likely to develop osteoarthritis, the most prevalent type of arthritis, as it affects their ability to absorb stress and maintain smooth joint movement.

Although osteoarthritis usually appears between the ages of 40 and 50, people with other types of arthritis or those with certain risk factors may experience it earlier. However, arthritis can strike people of any age, even younger ones. It is not just a condition that affects the elderly. Thus, it is imperative to identify and evaluate symptoms in people of all ages in order to guarantee prompt diagnosis and suitable treatment, hence reducing the adverse effects of arthritis on people's health and quality of life.

◆ Infection

Both bacterial and viral infections have the ability to cause joint inflammation and destruction, which makes infection a major factor in the onset of arthritis. Septic arthritis also referred to as joint infections, can result from several bacteria infiltrating the joint area and causing cartilage and synovial components to deteriorate.

In a similar vein, several viral infections have the ability to set off immune reactions that attack joint tissues, leading to inflammatory arthritis. People who have had repeated staph infections around a joint, multiple bouts of gout, or joint infections are more likely to develop arthritis. These infections can set off an inflammatory cascade that worsens joint damage and makes people more vulnerable to long-term arthritic diseases. In order to prevent long-term joint issues, infections might worsen pre-existing arthritis or cause flare-ups. This emphasizes the significance of early treatment and infection management methods.

◆ Autoimmune Factors

Rheumatoid arthritis, psoriatic arthritis, juvenile idiopathic arthritis, and lupus are examples of inflammatory arthritis in which the body's immune system attacks its tissues. What causes this needs to be clarified. However, it could be related to a variety of factors, such as genetic predisposition, infections, or environmental exposure. Your immune system becomes sensitized, producing antibodies that assault your joints and organs.

♦ Injury

Previous joint injury might leave abnormalities on the normal smooth joint surface. Prior injury undoubtedly contributes to the development of wrist arthritis, as the intricate bone and cartilage structure can be quickly undermined by impact or compression. Another example is arthritis induced by a tibial plateau fracture, in which a shattered piece of bone enters the knee joint's cartilage.

♦ Lifestyle Risk Factors

Some lifestyle choices can worsen the symptoms of some types of arthritis and increase the risk of getting others. Interestingly, the stress we place on our joints today could put us at risk for developing arthritis later. This includes factors that lead to the development and advancement of arthritis, such as being overweight, not exercising enough, having bad posture, and performing repeated motions that put unnecessary strain on the joints.

♦ Smoking

Smoking raises the likelihood of developing rheumatoid arthritis, makes the condition worse, and raises the possibility of developing additional health problems. It is believed that smoking induces immunological dysregulation and inflammation, which can accelerate the onset of rheumatoid arthritis and the degradation of joints in smokers. In addition, giving up smoking is crucial for lowering the disease's activity and improving the affected individuals' overall health.

♦   Obesity

Due to the fact that obesity increases the load on weight-bearing joints, especially the hips and knees, it has a major negative influence on joint health. Being overweight speeds up the degradation of joint tissues by causing inflammation and wear and tear. The development and progression of arthritis are significantly influenced by this increased mechanical strain, highlighting the significance of weight control in maintaining joint function and reducing the risk of arthritis.

♦   Sports

If a high-level sport causes injury to a bone or joint or includes blunt force impact, it may cause arthritis. This occurs in contact sports and sports like long-distance running that continuously stress a joint. Conversely, regular, mild exercise helps reduce the signs and progression of arthritis by strengthening the surrounding muscles of a joint and providing it with support.

♦   Genetics

Although genetics' exact role in the development of arthritis is still unknown, it is crucial, particularly in some cases. Different types of arthritis may have different heightened risks based on family history. For example, a significant genetic component is evident in psoriasis and psoriatic arthritis, as about 40% of those who suffer from these disorders have family relatives who also have them. It is essential to comprehend these genetic predispositions in order to evaluate each person's risk and, where practical, take preventive action.

♦ Foods and Medications

Certain food choices and medication can increase uric acid levels in gout arthritis patients, which can cause excruciating flare-ups. Purine-rich foods and drinks, such as beer, are generally advised to be avoided by those who have gout. It becomes crucial to regulate diet and medicine to avoid excessive uric acid accumulation in order to lower the risk of gout attacks. Gout management and reducing the frequency of debilitating flare-ups require the use of appropriate medication in addition to dietary modifications.

♦ Work Hazards

People who work in manual labor or engage in repetitive motion activities may be more susceptible to developing arthritis and joint damage. Protective measures are frequently used to reduce the incidence of joint injuries. These include ergonomic changes and safe lifting techniques. Workplace safety and preventive measures are crucial since even seemingly insignificant repetitive motions, like pushing carts or pulling levers, can eventually destroy bone and joint cartilage.

Arthritis develops as a complex process impacted by a number of variables. Even while many causes and risk factors, such as age and genetics, are unavoidable, proactive measures can be taken to lessen the risk and progression of arthritis. Sustaining a healthy weight, enforcing ergonomic working practices, and engaging in frequent physical exercise can all help safeguard joint health.

In addition, controlling underlying diseases like diabetes or obesity and abstaining from actions that worsen joint damage, including smoking, can significantly lower the risk of developing arthritis. Following treatment regimens and making lifestyle changes can help people with pre-existing diagnoses maintain joint function and slow the progression of their disease. People with arthritis can maximize long-term results and improve their quality of life by prioritizing preventive measures and following treatment plans.

The Role of Immune System in Autoimmune Arthritis Conditions

The term "autoimmune arthritis conditions" refers to a class of diseases marked by dysregulated immune responses, chronic inflammation, and joint damage. Clarifying the pathophysiology of these disorders, locating viable therapeutic targets, and creating efficient treatment plans all depend on understanding the immune system's function in them.

The term "autoimmune arthritis" refers to a set of illnesses in which the immune system incorrectly attacks the body's tissues, particularly the joints. The most common autoimmune arthritis disorders include SLE, JIA, PsA, and RA. These disorders have different clinical presentations and underlying genetic causes, but they are all marked by immune system abnormalities that result in persistent inflammation, synovial hyperplasia, and joint degradation.

The body's defense system against infections and foreign invaders is the immune system, which is made up of an intricate web of tissues, cells, and molecules. Normal conditions allow it to discriminate between self and non-self-antigens, eliciting the proper immune response to drive out pathogens while preserving tolerance to self-tissues. This self-tolerance is compromised in autoimmune diseases such as RA and PsA, though, and as a result, joint tissues are targeted by the production of inflammatory mediators and autoantibodies.

Pathogenesis of Autoimmune Arthritis

Multiple factors contribute to the pathogenesis of autoimmune arthritis. Environmental triggers, dysregulated immune responses, and genetic predisposition are all involved. Certain polymorphisms in genes encoding immune-related molecules and alleles of the human leukocyte antigen (HLA) confer genetic susceptibility. By causing aberrant immune activation and inflammation, environmental factors like infections, smoking, and hormonal changes can either cause or worsen autoimmune arthritis. The autoimmune arthritis is associated with synovial inflammation, cartilage degradation, and bone erosion. This is attributed to the dysregulation of T lymphocytes, B lymphocytes, and pro-inflammatory cytokines, specifically tumor necrosis factor-alpha (TNF-α), interleukin-1 (IL-1), and interleukin-6 (IL-6).

What Do T Cells Do in Autoimmune Arthritis?
How Do They Function?

T-cells are a subset of lymphocytes, which are white blood cells. They aid in the defense against illness and infection by your immune system. Two primary kinds exist. T-cells that are cytotoxic kill diseased cells. Helper T-cells function as messengers, directing other immune cells to combat infection.

From the bone marrow, T cells develop in the thymus. The thymus is a gland in the lymphatic system primarily responsible for promoting the maturation of mature T cells (thymus-derived is what the "T" in T cell lymphocyte means).

T cells are essential to the pathophysiology of autoimmune arthritis because they coordinate immune responses and maintain joint inflammation. CD4+. Th1 and Th17 subsets and regulatory T (Treg) cells are formed during differentiation of T helper (Th) cells and have different roles in autoimmune arthritis. Th1 cells stimulate synovial inflammation and macrophage activation by producing pro-inflammatory cytokines like interferon-gamma (IFN-γ). Conversely, Th17 cells cause tissue damage and neutrophil recruitment in the joints by secreting IL-17 and IL-21. The dysfunction of Treg cells in autoimmune arthritis exacerbates the severity of the disease by maintaining immune tolerance and suppressing excessive inflammation.

The Roles of B Cells and Autoantibodies

One subset of white blood cells called B cells, or B lymphocytes, is essential to the adaptive immune response. Antibodies are proteins that identify and neutralize particular pathogens, including bacteria, viruses, and toxins. Their main function is to produce these proteins. The bone marrow is the source of B cells, which develop there or in lymphoid organs like the spleen and lymph nodes.

The pathogenesis of autoimmune arthritis is influenced by B lymphocytes, which produce autoantibodies against self-antigens in the joints, including anti-citrullinated protein antibodies (ACPAs) and rheumatoid factor (RF). RF is a primary marker of RA, an autoantibody directed against the immunoglobulin G (IgG) Fc region. It is associated with both the severity and course of the disease. The formation of immune complexes, complement activation, and synovial inflammation are caused by ACPAs' recognition of citrullinated peptides derived from proteins found in joint tissues. With biologic medications like rituximab and belimumab proving effective in clinical trials, targeting B cells and autoantibodies has emerged as a viable therapeutic approach in autoimmune arthritis.

The Role of Innate Immunity in Autoimmune Arthritis

Inflammation in autoimmune arthritis is initiated and maintained in large part by innate immune cells, such as neutrophils, dendritic cells, and macrophages. After infiltrating the synovium, macrophages release reactive oxygen species (ROS), matrix metalloproteinases (MMPs), and pro-inflammatory cytokines that exacerbate tissue damage and joint degradation. As antigen-presenting cells in the synovial microenvironment, dendritic cells stimulate T cells and boost adaptive immune responses. After being drawn to the inflammatory joints, neutrophils release cytotoxic molecules and create neutrophil extracellular traps (NETs), exacerbating tissue damage and prolonging inflammation in autoimmune arthritis.

Inflammatory Pathways and Cytokine Signaling

In autoimmune arthritis, cytokines are crucial in modulating inflammatory reactions and tissue damage. IL-1, IL-6, and TNF-α are important pro-inflammatory cytokines linked to bone erosion, cartilage deterioration, and synovial inflammation. Biologic drugs that target these cytokines, like TNF inhibitors and IL-6 receptor antagonists, have entirely changed the way autoimmune arthritis is treated by reducing symptoms and stopping the disease's progression.

Additionally, the Janus kinase or signal transducer and activator of transcription (JAK/STAT) pathway and the nuclear factor-kappa B (NF-κB) pathway are possible therapeutic targets for the development of future medications. In autoimmune arthritis, these pathways play a crucial role in the cytokine generation process and immune cell activation.

The start and progression of autoimmune arthritis can be altered by environmental variables such as infections, smoking, nutrition, and stress that impact immune responses and inflammatory pathways.

Environmental factors that affect immune responses and inflammatory pathways, such as infections, smoking, diet, and stress, can modify the onset and course of autoimmune arthritis. In those who are vulnerable, infections—especially those caused by bacteria and viruses—can aggravate the symptoms of an autoimmune reaction and increase disease activity. One known risk factor for RA is smoking, which changes immune cell function and encourages protein citrullination, both of which contribute to the pathophysiology of the disease.

Diet and gut microbiota makeup play a significant role in autoimmune arthritis. Certain food components and microbial communities that impact immunological homeostasis and inflammation have an impact on the gut-joint axis. Psychosocial stressors and mental health issues can exacerbate autoimmune arthritis through the disruption of neuroendocrine pathways and the stimulation of systemic inflammation.

Future Perspectives and Therapeutic Approaches

The goal of treating autoimmune arthritis is to improve quality of life, maintain joint function, and reduce inflammation and joint damage while also reducing symptoms. Treatment options for autoimmune arthritis typically include corticosteroids, biologic agents, disease-modifying antirheumatic medications (DMARDs), and nonsteroidal anti-inflammatory drugs (NSAIDs). The patient's preferences, the condition's severity, and its clinical manifestations all influence the therapy option.

The method by which autoimmune arthritis is treated has radically changed as a result of medicines that target specific cytokines, immune cells, and signalling pathways, and they are safer and more effective than traditional DMARDs. New therapeutic modalities that promise to improve patient outcomes and treat autoimmune arthritis include immune modulation techniques, cell-based therapies, and small molecule inhibitors.

Joint damage, persistent inflammation, and dysregulated immune responses are the hallmarks of the complex and diverse group of diseases known as autoimmune arthritis. The immune system is crucial to the pathophysiology of these disorders because it initiates inflammatory cascades and sustains joint tissue damage. Creating focused, therapeutic interventions and individualized treatment plans requires understanding the immunological mechanisms underlying autoimmune arthritis. Through sustained research and cooperative endeavors, we can attain a more comprehensive comprehension and administration of autoimmune arthritis, ultimately augmenting the standard of living for those who endure these incapacitating ailments.

Chapter 2:
Types of Arthritis and Their Symptoms

The term "arthritis" refers to a broad range of conditions affecting your body's connective tissues, joints, and surrounding tissue. Although there are differences in symptoms, joint pain and stiffness are the most prevalent ones. When this pain happens, carrying out routine, everyday tasks can be challenging.

Over a hundred various conditions exist under the broad category of arthritis. The most prevalent kinds include osteoarthritis (OA), rheumatoid arthritis (RA), psoriatic arthritis (PsA), fibromyalgia, and gout. Many diseases, including arthritis, can cause excruciating pain in a variety of ways. The CDC has released worrisome figures that highlight the implications of arthritis. The results shed light on the wide-ranging implications of this illness, indicating its significant influence on people and society as a whole. The CDC's research highlights the critical need for increased awareness, early intervention, and effective management options to meet the challenges posed by arthritis. As a result, healthcare professionals, governments, and the general public must recognise the importance of these results and work together to develop proactive measures to reduce the impact of arthritis on people's health and well-being.

Approximately one-quarter of people with arthritis experience severe pain, defined as a score of seven or higher on a ten-point scale. Furthermore, more than one-third of individuals affected report significant difficulties in completing their personal and professional commitments. These findings highlight arthritis's severe impact on physical health and overall quality of life, emphasising the critical need for appropriate management measures to reduce its burdens.

Different treatments, both with and without medication, exist for the various types of arthritis pain. Different kinds of arthritis can indeed result in a range of pains, each with special traits and effects on different people. For instance, osteoarthritis (OA) frequently presents as a dull, excruciating pain in the afflicted joints, especially during or after activity. Over time, as the cartilage deteriorates and causes friction and inflammation between the bones, this kind of pain usually gets worse.

One of the common signs of osteoarthritis (OA) is stiffness in the joints, especially in the morning or after periods of inactivity. Depending on the areas affected by degenerative changes, osteoarthritis (OA) pain is typically localised to certain joints, such as the hands, spine, hips, or knees.

Let's look at the different kinds of arthritis, their signs and symptoms, the pain they cause, and ways to make them feel better.

❖ Osteoarthritis

Once upon a time, osteoarthritis (OA) was thought to be a "wear and tear" condition often associated with ageing. But now that we know, it affects all of the joint's components, including the bone, cartilage, ligaments, fat, and synovium—the tissue that lines the joint. Osteoarthritis damages cartilage changes the form of bones, and induces inflammation, which can result in pain, stiffness, and loss of movement.

While OA can impact any joint, it usually affects the hands, knees, hips, neck, and lower back. Although OA primarily affects people over 50, it can also strike those much younger, especially if they have experienced a previous joint injury like a meniscus or ACL tear. Usually, it takes a while to develop, but following an injury of this kind, it can happen in a matter of years. Not everyone ages will develop osteoarthritis (OA); some people do not.

Osteoarthritis causes painful and difficult joint movement as a result of the gradual degradation of the cartilage and fluid that protects the joint. Eventually, the joint's bones might rub against one another directly, causing excruciating pain. The process of osteoarthritis (OA), which most commonly affects the knees, hips, hands, and spine, also involves inflammation.

The following factors can raise your risk of developing osteoarthritis:

- Age: As people age, their muscles weaken, and their body's capacity for self-healing decreases. Osteoarthritis is not a necessary consequence of aging, though. Many live long lives devoid of symptoms of illness.
- Gender: Compared to men, women are more likely to develop osteoarthritis.
- Family history: Hand and finger osteoarthritis frequently runs in families, especially among women.
- Excess weight: Being overweight increases the strain on weight-bearing joints like the spine, hips, and knees and raises the possibility of injury. It is now believed that gut bacteria that thrive on fat also play a role in joint inflammation.
- Joint injury: Joints damaged by an accident or sports-related injury in the past may develop osteoarthritis. Reconstructive surgery, particularly knee surgery, can up the risk of osteoarthritis by seven times.

- Occupation: Excessive, repetitive physical activity can deteriorate joints and cause osteoarthritis. Some examples are professional athletes, dancers, farmers, and construction workers.
- Other joint conditions: Rheumatoid, gout, and septic arthritis are a few examples of arthritis that can occasionally harm joints. Osteoarthritis is also more common in people whose joints are malformed from birth or over time.

Symptoms of Osteoarthritis

- If any of the following symptoms persist for longer than two weeks, consult a physician:
- Joint stiffness following prolonged sitting or getting out of bed
- Joint pain, either during motion or while at rest
- Inflammation around the joint
- Weakness in the muscles
- Excruciating cracking or creaking when joints move.
- Diagnosis of osteoarthritis

Along with evaluating your symptoms, your doctor will perform a physical examination. It's critical to describe the precise location, duration, and impact of pain on your range of motion. In contrast to other disorders, osteoarthritis is not detectable by blood tests. Although osteoarthritis can be confirmed by X-rays and MRI scans, the results may not necessarily correspond to your degree of discomfort or function.

How to manage osteoarthritis

There is no known cure, but there are numerous strategies to manage your symptoms and lessen their influence on your daily life. You can take charge of your health and condition, but your health team will be there to guide you. Non-pharmacological approaches to managing osteoarthritis include the following:

i.   Exercise:

When you exercise properly, you can improve your flexibility and general fitness and reduce pain without endangering your joints. Aerobic, strengthening, and stretching exercises are crucial for:

- Preserving and returning normal range of motion in joints
- Lessening aches and stiffness
- Boosting your muscle mass
- Controlling your weight
- Boosting your vitality and wellbeing.

Walking, swimming, tai chi, and hydrotherapy are all beneficial types of exercise. Remember that commonplace pursuits like housework and gardening can serve as great sources of physical activity.

ii.   Heat and cold:

Heat can ease pain and stiffness in an arthritic joint by promoting blood circulation. Taking a hot shower first thing in the morning could help you prepare for the day. An inflamed joint will already feel warm; avoid applying heat to it. Instead, a cold pack should be used in the affected area to limit blood flow and lessen pain.

iii.   Joint protection:

You can use "gizmos and gadgets" to lessen the strain on your joints. Your feet, knees, hips, and back will benefit from the shock-absorbing properties of supportive, padded shoes. Reducing weight and stress on a sore hip or knee can be achieved by using a walking stick. Make changes to your living or working environment to cut down on pointless activities and adopt proper posture to ease the strain on your joints and muscles.

iv.   Stress-relief

Exhaustion and stress can exacerbate pain. Develop your ability to set priorities, pace yourself, and organize your day around what you can actually accomplish. Develop your relaxation skills to release the stress and discomfort from your body.

v.   Complementary therapies

Research indicates that while some complementary therapies and products can be helpful in managing osteoarthritis symptoms, others have not shown to be very effective. It is recommended that you speak with a licenced therapist, physician, or another specialist before starting any complementary product or therapy. Supplements for health may interfere with other prescriptions, and you may not get the same results as your friend.

vi.   Surgery

Surgery might be required to replace or repair a severely damaged joint. The most common joint replacements are those to the knee and hip. However, if osteoarthritis is well monitored and treated in its early stages, the need for "last resort" surgery may be avoided.

There is presently no recognised treatment for osteoarthritis; nevertheless, there are ways to manage the illness and lessen discomfort, like keeping up a good standard of life, staying mobile, and continuing physical activity.

❖ Rheumatoid Arthritis

Joint pain and inflammation are symptoms of rheumatoid arthritis (RA). It occurs when the synovium, the lining that lines the joints, is attacked by the immune system acting improperly. The disease frequently affects the hands, knees, or ankles, and it typically affects the same joint on both sides of the body, such as both hands or knees. However, there are instances when RA also results in issues with the heart, circulatory system, eyes, and/or lungs.

The hallmark of rheumatoid arthritis (RA) is a malfunctioning immune system that causes the body to mistakenly attack its tissues, especially the joints and other organs. In autoimmune diseases such as RA, inflammation becomes overactive. It targets healthy tissues, including the synovium lining the joints, in contrast to the immune system's normal response, which produces inflammation to protect against viruses, bacteria, and other invaders. Over time, this ongoing inflammation can exacerbate pain and discomfort by causing irreversible harm to joints and other organs.

A complex interaction between genetic predisposition, environmental triggers, and dysregulated immune responses leads to the pathogenesis of RA. Genetic factors, such as particular alleles of the human leukocyte antigen (HLA), are important in predisposing people to RA because they affect immune system function and susceptibility to environmental triggers. Infections, smoking, and hormonal changes are examples of environmental variables that can hasten the onset of RA or worsen disease activity by stimulating the immune system and sustaining inflammation.

RA causes dysregulation of a number of immune cells, including macrophages, T lymphocytes, and B lymphocytes, which prolongs tissue damage and inflammation. Activated T cells release pro-inflammatory cytokines, including as tumour necrosis factor-alpha (TNF-α), interleukin-1 (IL-1), and interleukin-6 (IL-6), which cause cartilage degradation, bone erosion, and synovial inflammation. Rheumatoid factor and anti-citrullinated protein antibodies (ACPAs) produced by B cells greatly aggravate tissue damage and the development of immune complexes in the joints. By quickening the inflammatory process and assisting in the breakdown of joint structures, these antibodies are essential to the pathophysiology of rheumatoid arthritis. They also promote immunological complex development, which worsens inflammation and tissue damage in the afflicted joints.

Synovial inflammation in RA creates an environment that is conducive to inflammatory cell recruitment and activation, which fuels the destructive cycle within the joint. The creation of pannus, synovial hyperplasia, and joint degeneration are caused by the release of various pro-inflammatory mediators, matrix metalloproteinases (MMPs), and tissue-destructive enzymes by synovial fibroblasts in response to inflammatory stimuli.

Apart from affecting joints, RA is a systemic illness that can impact various organs and systems across the body. Extra-articular symptoms of RA can include pulmonary symptoms like interstitial lung disease and pleuritis, as well as cardiovascular problems like accelerated atherosclerosis and an increased risk of myocardial infarction. Moreover, systemic inflammation in RA is linked to higher rates of osteoporosis, psychological comorbidities, and metabolic syndrome, highlighting the significance of comprehensive management plans that target the disease's extra-articular as well as articular manifestations.

Cause of Rheumatoid Arthritis (RA)

Honestly, the actual causes of rheumatoid arthritis are unknown, however, the following factors may increase the risk:

- Age: Rheumatoid arthritis can strike anyone at any time, although it usually appears between the ages of 25 and 50.
- Gender: The likelihood of RA in women is two to three times higher than in men.
- Family history: Certain genes have been connected to rheumatoid arthritis in certain individuals. That said, this does not guarantee you will get the illness.
- Hormones: Rheumatoid arthritis may develop as a result of hormonal changes that occur during and after pregnancy, during breastfeeding, and as a result of using oral contraceptives. They may also exacerbate or lessen symptoms.
- Smoking: Compared to nonsmokers, smokers have a higher incidence of rheumatoid arthritis.
- Infection: In individuals with genetic connections, infection may be the cause of RA. However, rheumatoid arthritis cannot be contracted or spread; it is not contagious.

Symptoms of Rheumatoid Arthritis

Rheumatoid arthritis usually starts slowly and affects the same joints on both sides of the body. In some people, it advances swiftly.

Here are a few rheumatoid arthritis symptoms:

- Soreness and edema in the wrists, fingers, or balls of the feet
- Waking up in the morning with stiffness
- Painful, swollen, and hot joints

- Fever, fatigue, decreased appetite, and reduction in body weight

Note: The effects of RA are unpredictable. Symptoms may appear and disappear with no discernible pattern, and you may experience flares. This is the moment when joints are most inflamed and painful.

Rheumatoid arthritis has varying effects on individuals. Some patients will experience flares followed by remissions. Only a few people will develop a severe type that causes considerable impairment and inflammation in other parts of their bodies, such as their eyes, skin, heart, lungs, or nerves.

Diagnosis of Rheumatoid Arthritis

Blood tests and X-rays allow your doctor to determine how quickly your arthritis is progressing. This determines the appropriate therapy to recommend and the expected future prognosis. You will then be referred to a rheumatologist. People who receive an early diagnosis and treatment are far more likely to avoid joint injury.

How to Manage Rheumatoid Arthritis

Like other kinds of arthritis, rheumatoid arthritis has no cure. The effect is different from person to person, so your doctor or rheumatologist will modify your treatment to your symptoms and severity. They may need to try many therapies to determine the best.

To prevent RA from taking over your life, you should engage in physical activity, work with your healthcare team, and use self-management techniques.

These non-medication therapies will help manage rheumatoid arthritis:

a. Exercise

Exercise is essential for managing arthritis and provides several physical and mental health benefits. By including a variety of exercise routines in your regimen, you can minimize pain and fatigue, build strength and flexibility, and boost overall vitality.

- Range of Motion Exercises: Range of motion Exercises are essential for keeping joints mobile and flexible. Incorporating gentle exercises that target all joints and encompass their full range of motion is essential. Consistent engagement in such exercises not only preserves joint flexibility but also wards off stiffness. Integrating these activities into your daily regimen not only safeguards joint health and mobility but also enhances overall physical well-being.

  Regular physical exercise is essential for maintaining proper joint function and general health. Individuals who incorporate workouts that improve flexibility and mobility can reduce their risk of joint stiffness while also improving their overall physical well-being. These exercises should be done on a daily basis to keep your joints healthy and mobile. Furthermore, adopting a range of workouts that focus on different muscle groups can give complete advantages while also improving general fitness and well-being. Individuals who include these exercises into their everyday regimen can successfully manage joint health while still maintaining an active lifestyle.

- Strengthening Exercises: Strengthening exercises help maintain muscular tone and preserve joints. These workouts stabilize joints and increase total functional capability by focusing on specific muscle groups. Incorporating resistance training and bodyweight movements into your workout program helps improve muscular strength and endurance.

- Stretching Exercises: Stretching exercises reduce discomfort and enhance flexibility in the muscles and tendons that surround joints. Stretching on a regular basis decreases stiffness, increases joint mobility, and minimises the risk of injury. Focus on modest, continuous stretches that target specific muscle groups affected by arthritis.

- Cardiovascular Exercises: Walking, swimming, and cycling have several benefits for those with rheumatoid arthritis. These low-impact workouts improve the heart, boost energy levels, and aid with weight management. Physical fitness and regular cardiovascular health can both be enhanced by regular cardiovascular exercise. Exercises with high impact, such as running or aerobics, should be avoided since they may exacerbate inflammation and pain in the joints. Regularly engaging in household tasks and gardening are excellent means of obtaining regular exercise. Pacing oneself is crucial to preventing excess and igniting a flare. Ask your physiotherapist what exercises are best for you.

- Hydrotherapy: Exercising in warm water offers a unique therapeutic approach for rheumatoid arthritis. Water's buoyancy decreases joint stress, allowing for moderate, low-impact motions. Exercising in warm water helps to ease pain and muscular tension and promotes relaxation. Consider adding hydrotherapy sessions into your fitness routine to reap the benefits of this relaxing and effective therapeutic method.

b.   Heat and cold

Heat and cold therapy are widely used to treat arthritis and other musculoskeletal disorders. Heat alleviates pain and stiffness, lessens muscular spasms and tightness, and improves range of motion. It works by increasing blood circulation, encouraging relaxation, and relieving aching muscles and joints. However, it is important to note that applying heat to an inflamed joint might worsen inflammation and suffering.

c.   Joint protection

Shoes with support and cushioning will act as shock absorbers for the back, hips, knees, and feet. 'Gizmos and gadgets, along with other practical strategies, could help you overcome daily obstacles, particularly when it comes to using your hands and fingers. Your occupational therapist can offer advice on minimizing fatigue, protecting your joints, and facilitating mobility.

d.   Stress-relief

Exhaustion and stress can exacerbate pain. Develop your ability to set priorities, pace yourself, and organize your day around what you can actually accomplish. Use relaxation techniques to reduce pain and tension.

Healthy Diets for Rheumatoid Arthritis

A nutritionally balanced diet not only provides energy to the body but also strengthens the immune system and preserves the integrity of bones and tissues. Fish oil, high in omega-3 fatty acids, has emerged as a crucial ally in the fight against inflammatory arthritis due to its powerful anti-inflammatory characteristics. Incorporating fish oil into one's diet can considerably reduce symptoms and improve joint health and well-being.

Some foods may cause a flare, while others may alleviate your symptoms, although this varies by individual.

Notably, no diet or supplement can cure rheumatoid arthritis; however, they can help manage the pain, and what works for others may not work for you. Be prepared to explore and consult with a licensed dietitian or your rheumatologist before starting a specific diet or using supplements.

Social And Emotional Support

Rheumatoid arthritis pain, which is unpredictable, can have a detrimental psychological and emotional influence on a person.

It is normal to feel fear, frustration, grief, and fury. Your health and welfare need you to accept and receive emotional support.

Surgery

Surgery may be required for people with rheumatoid arthritis. From minor interventions like tendon or nerve release to more involved operations like joint replacement, procedures come in a variety of forms. Though rare, surgical interventions can greatly reduce symptoms and enhance the quality of life for those afflicted.

❖ Juvenile idiopathic arthritis

Juvenile idiopathic arthritis (JIA) is the most prevalent kind of arthritis in children under the age of sixteen. It shows symptoms like stiffness, swelling, and ongoing joint pain. While some children may only have symptoms for a few months, others may have them for several years. Because JIA and its different subtypes are chronic, they can cause significant side effects like inflammation of the eyes, joint damage, and growth issues.

JIA is also an autoimmune disease, meaning that instead of the immune system's normal defense against infection, it mistakenly attacks healthy tissues, causing inflammation. Each person experiences JIA symptoms differently, and they can fluctuate from day to day and week to week. There may be sporadic "flares" in which symptoms worsen; the illness sometimes appears to temporarily go away.

In JIA, the immune system targets the synovium, a thin membrane lining the joints that secretes a fluid to promote easy mobility. As a result, the joints become painful and swollen. If inflammation is not controlled, it can harm bones, cartilage, and joints, as well as weaken the muscles that surround the joint.

Symptoms of Juvenile Idiopathic Arthritis Include:

- Joint pain: Prolonged soreness in one or more joints, frequently combined with tenderness.
- Joint swelling: An apparent enlargement caused by fluid buildup and inflammation in the afflicted joints.

- Joint stiffness: Specifically in the morning or after periods of inactivity, which is characterised by a restricted range of motion and difficulty moving the affected joints
- Fatigue: Chronic inflammation and interrupted sleep patterns can cause general fatigue and lethargy.
- Fever: Systemic symptoms may include fever, malaise, and rash, especially in instances with systemic JIA.

Causes Of Juvenile Idiopathic Arthritis

JIA is thought to be caused by a mix of genetic susceptibility, environmental factors, and dysregulated immunological responses, while the exact reasons remain unknown. Genetic factors, such as certain human leukocyte antigen (HLA) alleles, increase vulnerability to autoimmune illnesses like JIA. Infections, hormonal changes, and tobacco smoke exposure can all cause or worsen symptoms in genetically prone people. Immune cell dysregulation, including T lymphocytes, B lymphocytes, and macrophages, causes joint inflammation and tissue damage.

Subtypes Juvenile Arthritis

JIA has numerous subtypes, each with different characteristics. In general, they are all characterized by at least six weeks of joint pain, swelling, warmth, and stiffness. The JIA subtypes are as follows:

◊   Oligoarthritis, or oligoarticular JIA:

Oligoarthritis is the most prevalent subtype of JIA. It affects four or fewer joints, usually the larger ones like the elbows, knees, and ankles. Symptoms like joint pain, stiffness, and swelling are common. Although oligoarthritis may have a favorable prognosis, it can eventually spread to other joints. In addition to oligoarthritis, some children develop uveitis, an inflammation of the eyes that must be continuously watched and treated to minimise complications and preserve eyesight.

◊   Polyarthritis, or polyarticular JIA:

Five or more joints, mainly on both sides of the body, are affected by polyarthritis. Both big and small joints may be affected, including the fingers, wrists, knees, and toes. Polyarthritis affects about 25% of children with JIA. If left untreated, this subtype can result in severe joint inflammation, damage to the joints, and functional impairment. For kids with polyarthritis, symptom management and avoiding long-term complications require prompt diagnosis and vigorous treatment.

◊   Systemic JIA:

This particular form of JIA affects the entire body, including the skin, joints, and internal organs. Symptoms may include a high-pitching fever (103°F or more) that lasts at least two weeks, as well as rash, joint discomfort, and inflammation. Because systemic JIA affects the entire body and can produce major side effects such as liver, lung, or heart inflammation, it is particularly difficult to identify and treat. Typically, a combination of medicines is used to minimise inflammation and symptoms, along with close monitoring of organ function.

◊   Psoriatic JIA:

Joint symptoms may come first or later than skin symptoms. PsA can affect one or more joints, often involving the wrists, knees, ankles, fingers, or toes. Changes to the nails, such as pitting or detachment from the nail bed, may also occur. PsA therapy aims to minimise joint inflammation, manage skin complaints, and improve overall quality of life.

◊ Joint Infection-Related JIA:

Joint Infection-Related JIA or spondyloarthritis mainly affects the entheses—the places on the bone where muscles, ligaments, or tendons attach. Though it can also affect other areas like the fingers, elbows, pelvis, chest, and lower back, it usually affects the hips, knees, and feet. Enthesitis-related arthritis usually affects males more often and first appears in kids between the ages of eight and fifteen. For children with this subtype, prevention of joint injury and preservation of function depend on early identification and intervention.

◊ Undifferentiated JIA:

Undifferentiated arthritis is a subtype where symptoms do not fit perfectly into any defined categories, but inflammation is present in one or more joints. Over time, this subtype may evolve, eventually meeting the requirements for a specific subtype or staying undetected. To choose the best course of action for treatment and stop the condition from getting worse, constant observation and assessment are necessary.

Also, JIA symptoms can fluctuate. Flares are episodes of severe inflammation and deteriorating symptoms. Days or months may pass between flares.

Despite the difficulties this chronic condition presents, children with JIA can achieve better results and lead satisfying lives via cooperative efforts between healthcare practitioners, families, and support networks.

Diagnosis Juvenile Idiopathic Arthritis

Juvenile Idiopathic Arthritis cannot be diagnosed with a single test, and the waiting period for a diagnosis can be highly distressing for families. Your child will be referred to a physician who collaborates with a paediatric rheumatologist, an expert in treating arthritis in children.

The medical history, physical examination, blood tests, X-rays, and other testing will all be used to make the diagnosis. Some of these may need to be repeated in order to rule out other illnesses that cause joint pain and swelling.

How to Manage Idiopathic Juvenile Arthritis

JIA has no known cure but the remission (a state in which the disease exhibits little to no activity or symptoms) is conceivable. As soon as possible, the disease must be aggressively treated in order to bring it under control.

The objectives of JIA therapy are to:

- **Slow down or halt inflammation:** The goal is to stop more joint deterioration and related problems. In order to maintain joint integrity and function, this frequently entails the use of biological treatments, disease-modifying antirheumatic medications (DMARDs), or nonsteroidal anti-inflammatory medicines (NSAIDs) to suppress the immune response and reduce inflammation.
- **Relieve symptoms:** Relieving symptoms, controlling pain, and enhancing the overall quality of life are crucial aspects of JIA treatment. Physical therapy, assistive technology, and pain

management techniques are frequently used to reduce pain and enhance a child's capacity to engage in everyday activities and lead a more satisfying life.

- **Prevent joint and organ damage:** Preventing joint and organ damage is a crucial goal in JIA treatment, as chronic inflammation can lead to irreversible damage to joints and internal organs. Preserving the structural integrity of afflicted tissues and reducing the likelihood of long-term problems can be achieved with early intervention, suitable treatment, and routine monitoring.
- **Preserve joint function and mobility:** Maintaining mobility and joint function is crucial to reducing impairment and enhancing the child's independence. Physical and occupational treatments are frequently used with customized exercise regimens to maintain or improve joint range of motion, muscular strength, and total functional capability. This results in improved mobility and participation in daily activities.
- **Reduce long-term health effects:** Since JIA can have systemic effects in addition to joint inflammation, so reducing long-term health repercussions is essential to managing the condition. The effects of JIA on overall health and wellbeing can be lessened by close observation for any problems, such as growth abnormalities or inflammation of the eyes (uveitis), and with quick action as needed.
- **Achieve remission:** In JIA, achieving remission—typified by little or no disease activity and symptoms is the ultimate therapy objective. Many children with JIA can achieve remission, allowing them to lead active, productive lives with minimal interruption from the disease, with early diagnosis, aggressive treatment, and regular monitoring. Maintaining

remission and preventing disease flare-ups frequently need ongoing care and treatment plan adjustments.

The ultimate goal is for the family to live as much everyday life as possible with their child. The course of treatment will depend on your child's specific type of JIA, the affected joints, the severity of the condition, and how well your child tolerates the prescribed meds. Fortunately, most children will outgrow JIA with the right diagnosis and care. Therapy may not be necessary for around half of children with JIA as adults.

Treatment Methods:

1. Exercise

For children with JIA to be healthy and happy, parents must ensure they engage in physical exercise. Exercise maintains bones and muscles' strength, boosts confidence, and lessens JIA pain. You will need to locate sports and physical activities that your kid enjoys playing but that don't put them through too much discomfort. The physiotherapist for your kid might offer suggestions for appropriate workouts and activities. Swimming is pleasant and gives them freedom of movement, which makes it excellent!

Acupuncture and massage therapy are effective in reducing anxiety and stress in addition to pain. Acupuncture employs small needles put into the body at particular points to relieve pain. If the patient is afraid of needles, forceful pressure, known as acupressure, might be used in place of needles.

2. Rest

It's important that your child receives a good night's sleep and possibly some rest during the day because JIA can make them fatigued. Resting in bed all day does not constitute rest, as this might exacerbate stiffness and impair movement. There are various techniques to de-stress and cease thinking about your pain. These consist of deep breathing, visualization exercises, meditation, and reflecting back on pleasant experiences or serene locations. Certain distraction strategies may also help reduce pain in children with JIA, particularly during shot time. These consist of reading, being read to, coloring or drawing, and listening to music.

3. Nutritious diet

Children with JIA may have trouble eating, so it's critical to make sure they're getting enough food to maintain a good weight and energy level. Having a well-balanced diet is very important for your overall wellness. It is also crucial to include plenty of fresh fruits and calcium-rich dairy items like cheese, milk, and yoghurt. These foods include essential nutrients that support bone health, muscular function, and general well-being.

High-fat, sugary, and processed foods are among the foods that children with JIA should limit or stay away from because they can worsen the symptoms.

Supplement use in children is rarely studied. However, certain supplements taken by adults may also benefit kids. These include supplements containing omega-3 fish oil, which may help with stiffness and joint pain, and curcumin, a chemical present in turmeric. Strong bones can be developed by consuming calcium and vitamin D. Consult your child's doctor about vitamins and supplements. Some drugs have the potential to interact with other medicines and cause side effects.

4.   Managing flare-ups and pain

Infections, stressful times, or changes in medication can all cause flares, but they can also occur for no apparent reason at all. Your child may experience increased pain, stiff and swollen joints, and fatigue but difficulty falling asleep during a flare-up. This could impact their mood, creating a vicious cycle of suffering.

To help your kid during a flare-up, you can provide them with coping mechanisms like deep breathing exercises and relaxation techniques. You can also experiment with hot and cold packs, stretching exercises, massages, and distraction.

5.   Social and emotional support

JIA can provide difficulties for siblings, other family members, you, and your child. Explaining what happens during a flare may be challenging, so managing your child's arthritis as a team, with assistance from friends, family, and teachers, will be beneficial.

6.   Heat and Cold Therapies

The greatest therapies for sore joints and fatigued muscles are heat-based, such as heat pads or warm baths. For acute discomfort, cold is the best. It can lessen inflammation and numb sore places. Despite the difficulties this chronic condition presents, children with JIA can achieve better results and lead satisfying lives via cooperative efforts between healthcare practitioners, families, and support networks.

❖ Psoriatic Arthritis

Some persons with psoriasis (a disorder marked by the rapid proliferation of skin cells) may develop psoriatic arthritis, an inflammatory form of arthritis. It's an autoimmune condition, meaning your immune system mistakenly attacks healthy tissue. Patients with psoriatic arthritis experience problems with both their skin and joints. Symptoms could change according to the circumstances.

Skin problems typically appear first, followed by arthritis. However, psoriasis is not always present when joint issues arise. Although there isn't a treatment for psoriatic arthritis, there are several ways to minimise joint damage and discomfort.

About ten to thirty percent of those with the skin condition will also get psoriatic arthritis, which can affect one or more joints and range in severity from mild to severe. Some persons with arthritic symptoms never get psoriasis, while other times, joint issues manifest before the skin disease.

The majority of instances of psoriatic arthritis develop in adulthood and affect both men and women equally. Because the ailment affects people differently, it is readily confused with other types of arthritis.

Signs and Symptoms of Psoriatic Arthritis

Psoriatic arthritis can induce a variety of symptoms. Only some people with the condition have the same problems, and some have more serious ones than others. Symptoms could include:

Psoriatic arthritis symptoms can appear in a variety of ways, such as sausage-like swelling in fingers or toes, hand deformities, and discomfort in the feet, neck, or spine. Affected joints may stiffen and become painful, with surrounding tissues showing redness, heat, or edoema. Individuals may also experience red, scaly skin spots, itching, burning, and nail irregularities such as cracking or pitting. Common symptoms include pain and blurred vision in the eyes, as well as reduced range of motion and difficulty bending joints. Psoriatic arthritis patients frequently experience fatigue, which is influenced by a number of conditions in addition to pain and disease activity.

The actual etiology of psoriatic arthritis is unknown. However, medical professionals know it results from the body's immune system attacking healthy tissue. Once the joints get inflamed, then the skin produces too many cells due to this flawed process. Experts surmise that a combination of hereditary and environmental factors could cause immune system dysfunction in this regard.

Causes

Certain factors that may increase your risk are as follows:

- Having Psoriasis: The highest risk factor for psoriatic arthritis is having a diagnosis of psoriasis.
- Family History: Roughly 40% of those with psoriatic arthritis have psoriasis or arthritis in a family relative.
- An Infection: Infections with bacteria or viruses have the potential to stimulate the immune system and cause psoriatic arthritis in certain individuals.
- Age: Psoriatic arthritis can strike anyone, but it most frequently affects those in the 30 to 50 age range.
- Obesity: Carrying more weight strains tendons, increasing the risk of inflammation and psoriatic arthritis.

Treating and Managing Psoriatic Arthritis

Psoriatic arthritis (PsA) affects the skin and joints, making the treatment difficult. Medication and non-pharmacological therapy, like massage, exercise, and temperature-based interventions, can be combined in the treatment of PsA. The treatment strategy is structured to each patient's different symptoms and the disease's severity. The main goal of psoriatic arthritis treatment includes:

- Remission of the disease.
- A slower rate of disease progression.
- The relief of pain and related symptoms.
- Protection of the joints and epidermis

When treating joint problems, a multidisciplinary approach is frequently necessary, involving experts such as dermatologists for skin complaints and rheumatologists for joint problems. Working with a medical team enables a treatment plan to be designed to meet the patient's requirements.

The contributions of physical and occupational therapists are substantial; they offer structured exercises, methods for increasing joint flexibility and strength, and approaches for making daily tasks less painful. It is necessary to consult your healthcare providers before beginning any fitness regimen to ensure a safe and efficient strategy to control psoriatic arthritis.

An important component of controlling PsA is physical therapy and exercise. Frequent exercise increases general health, improves energy, improves mood, and relieves stiffness and pain. The suggested fitness program includes Stretching and strength training, along with low-impact cardiovascular activities like swimming, cycling, and walking.

a. Lifestyle Modifications

Preserve Your Energy: One of the most prevalent symptoms of juvenile idiopathic arthritis (JIA) is fatigue, which frequently affects daily functioning and quality of life. The key to efficiently managing fatigue is to schedule and pace your activities throughout the day. This entails setting priorities, dividing work into smaller, more manageable chunks, and scheduling enough time for rest and leisure. Making sure you get enough good-quality, long-lasting sleep is also essential for preventing JIA-related fatigue. By implementing these tactics, people can reduce tiredness, preserve energy, and lead more balanced lives.

b. Protect Your Joints

Daily activities can put stress on inflammatory joints, making them worse and perhaps causing more damage. People with joint integrity issues (JIA) can reduce this risk by altering their task performance or using devices and assistance that promote joint function. For example, employing assistive devices, adaptive equipment, or ergonomic tools can help lessen joint stress and discomfort, enabling people to perform daily tasks more efficiently and independently while maintaining joint integrity long-term.

c. Practice relaxation

JIA symptoms can be made worse by stress and tense muscles, which can lead to flare-ups and exacerbation of pain. By reducing these consequences, relaxation training can enhance mental and physical health. Methods that efficiently lower stress levels, promote tranquilly, and ease muscle tension include progressive muscle relaxation, yoga, deep breathing exercises, and mindfulness meditation. Through the integration of these techniques into their daily routines, people with JIA can enhance their coping strategies, effectively manage stress, and potentially lessen the frequency and intensity of flare-ups of their disease.

d. Avoid Smoking

Smoking raises your chance of heart disease, lung issues, and autoimmune diseases like psoriatic arthritis, among other health problems. People with JIA are more likely to acquire comorbidities such as high blood pressure, increased cholesterol, obesity, and diabetes, particularly if they have the psoriatic subtype. Smoking increases the likelihood of these problems by exacerbating joint discomfort and systemic inflammation. Thus, in order to improve overall health outcomes, slow the advancement of the disease, and reduce related consequences in people with JIA, quitting smoking is essential.

e. Healthy Eating

Eating a balanced diet is extremely important for general health and wellness, even if particular dietary therapies for juvenile idiopathic arthritis (JIA) are currently being discussed. In addition to providing vital nutrients and bolstering immune system performance, a diet high in fruits, vegetables, lean meats, and whole grains also helps reduce inflammation and maximise energy.

A healthy weight also lessens the strain on joints, relieving discomfort and increasing range of motion. People with JIA can improve their general health and possibly lessen the severity of their disease, as well as maximize the benefits of treatment by implementing appropriate eating habits.

f. Supplements

It's still being determined if supplements that have been researched to help with psoriatic arthritis symptoms or disease activity truly have any effect. Pilot trials have been conducted. However, most of them haven't been able to provide much information because of the study design, specifically the small sample size, brief length, and inadequate blinding. In a trial design, blinding occurs when neither the person administering the therapy nor the person receiving it is aware of whether they are administering or receiving the treatment under test or the placebo. Finding a valid conclusion about a study depends in large part on blinding.

g. Emotional and social assistance

Any chronic illness can negatively affect relationships, employment, social life, mood, and confidence. If you want to meet other people who have psoriatic arthritis, get in touch with a support group. You can also discuss how your family, friends, and medical team can best help you.

❖ Gout arthritis

As an inflammatory arthritis, gout does not produce systemic inflammation like RA or PsA. The issue with gout is elevated uric acid levels. Hyperuricemia, or elevated blood levels of uric acid, can occur when the body creates excessive amounts of uric acid or when the excess is not eliminated quickly enough, leading to uric acid crystals in joints. This causes inflammation in the joints that hurts excruciatingly.

If left untreated, these crystals may develop into lumps (tophi) in the tissues around the afflicted joints. Gout typically manifests abruptly, most frequently in the big toe's major joint but occasionally in other joints as well. You can feel good going to bed and wake up in severe pain when you have a flare-up of gout.

Many people assume that binge eating and excessive alcohol intake are the causes of gout arthritis. However, this is not the case. The major cause of elevated uric acid levels in your blood is your body's inability to eliminate it correctly. This might be due to genetics, weight, or pre-existing renal conditions.

Causes

Gout arthritis is caused by several causes, including:

- **Family history:** Some people have genes that limit their bodies' capacity to remove uric acid. Although not every family member will develop gout arthritis, the disease runs in families, and some people develop gout arthritis despite having no family history.
- **Excess weight:** Obesity and overweight impede the kidneys' ability to eliminate uric acid.
- **Age:** Gout attacks can occur in teenagers, but it typically strikes men over 40 and women after menopause.
- **Medications:** Diuretics or water pills might lessen the kidney's capacity to remove uric acid from the blood.
- **Other conditions:** Risk factors for gout arthritis include renal disease, high blood pressure, high blood sugar, and high cholesterol.

Purines are naturally occurring molecules found in all cells; the body breaks them down to produce gout in some persons with high uric acid levels. Purines may be found in a wide range of meals and beverages, including red meat, organ meats, shellfish, and sugar-filled beverages like beer.

Uric acid can form needle-like crystals that lodge in joints and cause sudden, severe pain and swelling. This can happen when uric acid builds up in the body due to too much purine-rich meal consumption or insufficient renal excretion.

Gout episodes, whether or not they are treated, typically reach their climax 12 to 24 hours later and then gradually subside on their own. Gout attacks can happen only once in a lifetime or sometimes every several years. If left untreated, recurrent bouts of gout can affect more joints, linger longer, and worsen over time. Large masses of uric acid crystals called tophi, which can eventually grow in soft tissues or the bones around joints and seem like hard lumps, can happen to some people.

Diagnoses

Effective gout management depends on monitoring uric acid levels. Accurate measurements may be obtained with a simple blood test that involves poking your thumb. To lessen the chance of gout attacks, uric acid levels should ideally be kept below 0.36 millimoles per litre (mmol/L). At least one annual blood test is necessary to monitor uric acid levels and provide prompt actions to avoid flare-ups.

Another method of diagnosing gout arthritis is to look for urate crystals in a sample of the fluid surrounding the joint. X-rays are not helpful for diagnosing the condition because they are frequently normal in the early stages but will reveal joint deterioration in later stages.

Treatments

Gout episodes do not have to be painful for you. You can manage gout arthritis and avoid kidney and joint damage by following your doctor's prescriptions for medication and moderation in food and drink.

The following techniques will be very helpful:

Gout medication: Gout medications fall into two categories: those that lower uric acid levels and those that address gout flare-ups. It is recommended to take uric acid medications daily, even in the absence of gout attacks.

Preventing gout in the joints: Even the pressure of sheets and blankets can be excruciating during a gout attack. To relieve your sore joints:

- Place something under the bedcovers and sit where people won't bump into you.
- Maintain the sore joint elevated and try using an ice pack.
- When experiencing a gout attack, stay still and take it easy until your symptoms subside.

Eating a balanced diet to prevent gout: One of the best ways to cure gout arthritis if you are overweight is to lose a few kg at a time. Certain food avoidance can help reduce blood uric acid levels and ward off gout attacks. Certain foods may cause a gout attack for you, although this varies from person to person.

- Eat three meals a day. Gout attacks can be triggered by starvation or overindulgence.
- Reduce your meat, poultry, and shellfish intake because they are high in purines.
- Take fruits, vegetables, and low-fat dairy products every day.

- Reduce your alcohol intake. Beer has more purines than other forms of alcohol, which increases the risk of gout attacks.
- Sip six to eight glasses of water daily and steer clear of sugar-filled beverages.

Footwear: Putting on shoes, or walking can be difficult if you have gout in your feet. Old shoes, slippers, jandals, and sandals need to provide more support for your feet and can throw off your balance. The appropriate shoes will be cozy and guard against additional joint deterioration. Shoes should have enough leeway (not too tight) if your foot swells. So, opt for:

- A wide toe
- An adjustable fit for the shoe using laces or Velcro
- A supportive, cushioned insole for your foot
- A tiny heel—high heels can cause issues for your knees, legs, and feet—- A deep heel to ensure that your foot fits appropriately in the shoe
- A sturdy, unworn-down sole.

Support: Make sure everyone in your family knows what to do in the case of a gout attack, and discuss with them how they can help you avoid gout arthritis by eating foods that will prevent gout and getting enough exercise. Encourage others who exhibit gout symptoms to seek treatment, as the condition may run in your family. By doing routine blood work and keeping an eye on your medication, your doctor will work with you to develop a plan for effectively managing your gout. Together, you can overcome gout arthritis and spare yourself or your loved ones needless misery.

❖ Lupus Arthritis

Lupus Arthritis is a chronic inflammatory condition in which the immune system attacks its own tissues and organs. Lupus-related inflammation damages the skin, joints, kidneys, brain, blood, heart, and lungs, among other internal organs.

Systemic lupus erythematosus is the most prevalent type of lupus (SLE). Although symptoms might vary widely, skin and joints are frequently affected. Organs like the brain, kidneys, and lungs could be impacted.

Other types of lupus include:

- **Discoid lupus:** This is characterized by a severe red rash that gets worse in the sun.
- **Cutaneous lupus:** Its severity varies, and it solely affects the skin.
- **Drug-induced lupus:** When using some drugs, people may develop lupus symptoms that disappear when they stop taking them.
- **Neonatal lupus:** This kind impacts the children of lupus-affected women. After delivery, skin symptoms typically disappear in a few weeks to months. Heart issues could result from it.

Causes of Lupus Arthritis

There is no known cause of lupus. Researchers believe that environmental factors like stress, viral infections, medications, or frequent exposure to potentially harmful chemicals can trigger persons with specific genes. Hormones may be involved because women with lupus frequently develop the disease during their reproductive years.

Signs and Diagnoses

Due to its tendency to mimic other disorders' signs and symptoms, lupus can be challenging to diagnose. Its symptoms can appear and disappear. Some people experience minor symptoms that gradually worsen. Others experience an abrupt onset of severe, sometimes fatal symptoms. The most typical ones consist of:

- Pain in the joints.
- Rash in the shape of a butterfly (on cheeks and nose).
- Fatigue.
- Mouth sores (usually without pain).
- Headaches.
- Sensitivity to light (both artificial and solar).
- Breathing difficulties or chest pain.

How to Manage or Control lupus

Lupus is unpredictable and varies from person to person. It has no known curr. Most people can manage it successfully with medication, lifestyle modifications, and team support from their healthcare provider.

Modification of Lifestyle

Making lifestyle adjustments can help you feel better, decrease symptoms, and lessen the chance of flare-ups. These consist of:

- Avoid smoking

- Applying sunscreen helps protect skin from the sun and avoid rashes
- Exercise frequently to avoid weariness and muscle weakness
- Rest; lower stress levels
- Eat a nutritious, well-balanced diet
- Enlist the help of loved ones, friends, healthcare providers, and support groups.

Flares

There are times when lupus patients experience minimal, silent symptoms or none at all. Sometimes, symptoms may be controlled for a period by medication or the nature of the condition, but other times, they may resurface. What triggers a flare-up in one individual might not be the same for another.

Being aware of your triggers can help you avoid flare-ups or lessen their severity. You and your physician can maintain the most excellent possible control over your illness by keeping track of your flares. Maintain a journal of your lupus symptoms, noting any activities or events prior to a flare-up.

Self-Care

Fruits, vegetables, whole grains, low-fat dairy, lean protein, and healthy fats like avocado and extra-virgin olive oil are all important components of a balanced diet. Opt for foods rich in omega-3s, as they have anti-inflammatory properties.

Resting helps to relieve inflammation and weariness when a disease is active, and joints are sore, swollen, or stiff. Frequent exercise can help reduce tension and pain when disease activity is low. Exercises for flexibility, muscular building, and low-impact aerobic activity are all part of a well-rounded program.

Skin rashes or flare-ups can result from ultraviolet (UV) radiation emitted by fluorescent lights or the sun. Use sunscreen with an SPF of 30 or greater at all times, and reapply it every hour or after swimming, perspiring, or changing clothes. Stay indoors between 10 a.m. and 4 p.m. when UV radiation is at its highest. Wear caps and protective apparel, and exercise extra caution if taking any medications that make you more photosensitive.

One typical symptom of lupus is fatigue. It's critical to pace oneself to avoid excessive fatigue ruining your day. Getting a good night's sleep might help prevent fatigue.

To have emotional support for navigating the ups and downs of a chronic illness:

- Build strong, healthy connections. Practice techniques that help lower your stress levels, such as breathing deeply, yoga, and meditation.
- Maintain your involvement in the things you enjoy doing to lift your spirits.
- Smoking damages the body and exacerbates the symptoms of lupus. Seek expert assistance if quitting is difficult for you on your own.

❖ Fibromyalgia

Fibromyalgia is a challenging and sometimes misunderstood disorder that appears largely as widespread pain and persistent tiredness, severely affecting the lives of people affected. While it has certain symptoms in common with arthritis, such as joint and muscular pain, medical specialists classify it as a pain disease. Unlike certain life-threatening disorders, fibromyalgia does not pose an immediate threat to one's physical health.

Still, its persistent symptoms can significantly affect several aspects of everyday living, including sleep quality and cognitive function. Furthermore, patients with fibromyalgia frequently have emotional difficulties, with research revealing a greater frequency of sadness and chronic anxiety among them. This emphasises the significance of using alternative treatments and seeking professional help to manage both the mental and physical symptoms of fibromyalgia.

Fibromyalgia's challenging nature sometimes leads to misconceptions and incorrect diagnoses, especially because its symptoms may resemble those of arthritis and other musculoskeletal disorders. Fibromyalgia, on the other hand, has been classified as a different pain condition because of its widespread and chronic nature. Fibromyalgia, unlike arthritis, which predominantly affects the joints, spreads to the muscles and soft tissues, causing widespread constant excruciating pain. This significant distinction emphasises the need for correct diagnosis and appropriate treatment methods in effectively addressing the particular problems offered by fibromyalgia.

The tremendous impact that fibromyalgia has on many aspects of everyday living cannot be overstated, even though it may not immediately cause a threat to life. Fibromyalgia patients' quality of life can be negatively impacted by their constant pain and exhaustion, which can make even simple chores difficult. A constant state of weariness and pain is created by sleep problems, a defining characteristic of the illness that worsens the mental and physical side effects. It can also be difficult to manage everyday tasks and activities due to the cognitive symptoms of fibromyalgia, sometimes known as "fibro fog," which can affect memory, focus, and general mental clarity.

In addition to physical symptoms, fibromyalgia is usually associated with emotional pain, with studies revealing a higher frequency of depression and persistent anxiety among individuals affected. The interaction between physical pain and emotional wellbeing emphasises the significance of taking a complete strategy to care, addressing both the physical and psychological elements of the condition.

Causes

The exact cause of fibromyalgia is not known. Researchers believe individuals with specific genes are impacted by a trigger (such as physical or mental stress or sickness). The pain impulses sent through their central nervous system (brain and spinal cord) are then amplified to an excessive degree, a condition known as centralised pain. That is why persons with fibromyalgia are more sensitive to pressure, heat, sound, and light than those without the disorder.

Fibromyalgia develops as a result of a complex interaction of genetic predisposition and environmental circumstances. Genetic susceptibility plays a key role, with research linking familial clustering and genetic markers to higher risk. However, the development of fibromyalgia is often preceded by a triggering event, which might differ greatly across individuals. Physical events, such as accidents or injuries; mental stresses, such as trauma or significant life changes; and specific diseases or infections have all been identified as possible causes.

Also, fibromyalgia has been linked to dysfunctions in neurotransmitter networks, notably those involving serotonin, dopamine, and norepinephrine. These neurotransmitters modulate pain perception, mood control, and stress responses, impacting the development and maintenance of fibromyalgia symptoms.

Fibromyalgia is a complicated condition with multiple triggers. While genetic predisposition is the starting point, environmental triggers and neurobiological changes drive the condition's growth and evolution. More study into the underlying processes is required to elucidate the specific aetiology of fibromyalgia and inform the development of focused therapy methods aimed at relieving symptoms and enhancing the quality of life for afflicted persons.

Symptoms

Fibromyalgia symptoms are similar to those of the severe flu, with sufferers suffering from tiredness, widespread pain, and cognitive fog. Fibromyalgia patients frequently describe their disease as being identical to fighting a never-ending sickness, with each day seeming like an uphill battle against crushing exhaustion, physiological discomfort, and mental fogginess. The tiredness is not just physical; it often goes deep, leaving people feeling spent and depleted despite their best attempts to rest and recover.

Similarly, the pain associated with fibromyalgia goes beyond localised discomfort, emerging as a diffuse agony that appears to pervade every part of the body. Chronic pain may be devastating, making even ordinary chores seem impossible. Furthermore, cognitive symptoms such as difficulties concentrating, memory lapses, and poor decision-making exacerbate the burden of fibromyalgia, leaving people feeling mentally foggy and confused. Overall, fibromyalgia symptoms may have a significant influence on all parts of a person's life, from physical health to cognitive function, and knowing the severity of these symptoms is critical for appropriate management and support.

- Pain and tenderness

Pain can sometimes start in one location, such as the neck and shoulders, and progress to other areas over time. The discomfort occurs on both sides of the body, above and below the waist. It may be minor or severe. Another characteristic of fibromyalgia pain is sensitivity to touch (tenderness). The American College of Rheumatology found 18 "tender points" (9 pairs) on the body that are extremely sensitive to touch in patients with fibromyalgia.

Pain has been characterised as searing, aching, stabbing, tingling, throbbing, soreness, or numbness (loss of sensation). It can vary depending on the time of day, exercise intensity, weather (particularly cold or wet environments), sleep habits, and stress. Although the discomfort may come and go, some people say it is constantly there.

- Fatigue and sleep challenges.

Sleep difficulties differ from person to person. Some people have trouble falling asleep or wake up often throughout the night. Others wake up feeling unrefreshed, even after sleeping all night. According to studies, a lack of sleep might exacerbate discomfort. These symptoms might lead to confusion between fibromyalgia and chronic fatigue syndrome (CFS).

Some individuals with fibromyalgia have poor energy levels and are constantly weary. Fatigue might be significant, causing more problems than pain.

- Memory and Thinking Problems

The notion of "fibro fog" is commonly used to denote the inability to pay attention or complete simple mental activities and forgetfulness or bad judgement.

These issues can arise and disappear anytime, but they are particularly common when someone is anxious or exhausted. Fibromyalgia patients may experience difficulties in learning, understanding, and remembering.

Diagnosis

Fibromyalgia is diagnosed mostly by a complete assessment rather than laboratory testing. This procedure consists of several critical components, including a full medical history, a comprehensive physical examination, and a careful assessment of symptoms. Here's a deeper look at the diagnostic criteria and evaluation procedure:

1. Medical History: The healthcare professional will get a thorough medical history, including questions about the patient's symptoms, onset, duration, and severity. They will ask about any prior medical illnesses, injuries, surgeries, or treatments that might be related to the present symptoms. In addition, the doctor will look into the patient's family history of medical illnesses like fibromyalgia or other chronic pain diseases.

2. Physical Examination: A physical examination is required to identify tenderness, pain, and other physical symptoms linked with fibromyalgia. The doctor will do a thorough exam, giving special attention to parts of the body that are known to be delicate in people with fibromyalgia. The Widespread Pain Index (WPI) identifies 19 unique painful locations.

3. Symptom Evaluation: Besides examining sensitive spots, the healthcare professional will examine the intensity and effect of fibromyalgia-related symptoms. Symptoms may include:

- Persistent fatigue that does not improve with rest or sleep.
- Disrupted sleep patterns, such as difficulties falling, staying asleep, or non-restorative sleep.
- Cognitive Dysfunction: Problems with memory, focus, and attention, sometimes known as "fibro fog."
- Other physical symptoms include headaches, muscular weakness, dizziness, numbness or tingling feelings, gastrointestinal disorders (e.g., irritable bowel syndrome), and hair loss.

4. Scoring System: To help with diagnosis, healthcare practitioners may use a scoring system based on WPI and symptom severity. The WPI measures pain and tenderness in 19 particular locations of the body, whereas the Symptom intensity (SS) score rates the intensity of accompanying symptoms on a scale of 0 to 3. These ratings serve to assess the severity and effect of fibromyalgia symptoms.

5. Symptom Duration: Symptoms must last at least three months to satisfy diagnostic criteria. This length distinguishes fibromyalgia from transitory or acute illnesses.

6. Exclusion of Other disorders: Although there are no particular laboratory tests for diagnosing fibromyalgia, healthcare practitioners may run blood tests and imaging procedures (e.g., X-rays) to rule out other disorders that may cause or contribute to persistent pain and exhaustion. These tests can help rule out underlying medical diseases such as autoimmune illnesses, thyroid abnormalities, and inflammatory arthritis.

In a nutshell, diagnosing fibromyalgia necessitates a thorough approach that takes into account the patient's medical history, physical examination results, symptom presentation, and the elimination of other possible causes of persistent pain and exhaustion. Collaboration between the patient and the healthcare professional is critical for the correct diagnosis and management of fibromyalgia.

Treatment

Fibromyalgia treatment focuses on symptom management and overall quality of life. Despite the fact that there is no known cure for fibromyalgia, there are several therapeutic options available to manage pain, exhaustion, sleep difficulties, and mental wellbeing. Medications, therapy, lifestyle changes, and self-care behaviours are frequently used in this strategy.

    i.   Multidisciplinary Approach:

Managing fibromyalgia sometimes involves collaboration among healthcare providers. This team might comprise a general care physician, a rheumatologist, a physical therapist, and a mental health expert. Each member plays an important role in meeting the different demands of fibromyalgia patients and personalising treatment regimens to individual needs.

    ii.   Medication:

A number of medicines have been licenced for fibromyalgia therapy. These medications function by modifying neurotransmitter levels in the brain, which aids in the regulation of pain perception. Some are targeting brain chemicals involved in pain processing. Other drugs, including anti-inflammatories, antidepressants, and sleep aids, may be administered to treat fibromyalgia-related pain, enhance sleep quality, and address mood disorders.

iii.   Cognitive Behavioural Therapy (CBT)

Cognitive Behavioural Therapy (CBT) is a highly effective treatment for fibromyalgia symptoms. Individuals can learn to recognise and fight harmful thinking patterns and behaviours that lead to pain and dysfunction by meeting with a skilled mental health counsellor. CBT seeks to create positive coping methods, increase relaxation abilities, and improve general psychological wellbeing.

iv.   Relaxation Techniques:

Deep breathing exercises, gradual relaxation of the muscles, and guided imagery are effective relaxation techniques that reduce muscular tension and discomfort and produce calm. Massage treatment is another effective complementary therapy that improves physical and emotional wellbeing by reducing muscular stiffness and increasing circulation.

v.   Mindfulness and Meditation Practices:

Mindfulness-based practices aim to cultivate present-moment awareness and acceptance of one's experiences. These techniques, such as mindfulness meditation and body scanning, can help people develop a nonjudgmental attitude towards pain and build resilience in dealing with fibromyalgia symptoms.

vi.   Exercise:

Exercising can help manage fibromyalgia by reducing pain, improving sleep quality, improving physical functioning, and boosting mood. Walking, swimming, and tai chi are all low-impact workouts that can provide considerable advantages. Contact a healthcare physician before beginning any exercise programme to ensure safety and appropriateness.

vii.   Self-Care Practices:

Self-care is essential for controlling fibromyalgia symptoms and improving overall wellbeing. Adequate sleep hygiene, stress reduction strategies, and a balanced lifestyle that includes nutritious eating habits, frequent exercise, limited alcohol intake, and smoking cessation are essential. Individuals with fibromyalgia can improve their physical and mental wellbeing by prioritising self-care.

The Progression and Prognosis of Various Arthritis Conditions

Understanding the progression and prognosis of diverse arthritis disorders is imperative for efficient administration and patient care. As we all know, a wide range of musculoskeletal conditions are included in the term "arthritis," defined by inflammation of the joints, which causes pain, stiffness, swelling, and a reduction in range of motion. The prognosis and progression of each form of arthritis are determined by its distinct traits, disease processes, and clinical manifestations. The progression and prognosis for seven common arthritic diseases are as follows:

Osteoarthritis (OA)

> **Progression:** The progressive degeneration of joint cartilage and underlying bone, which causes joint pain, stiffness, and functional impairment, is the hallmark of osteoarthritis. The symptoms of osteoarthritis (OA) usually develop over several

years as the illness progresses. People may initially have sporadic joint pain and stiffness, especially following extended periods of inactivity or overuse of the injured joint. Joint deformity, loss of function, and reduced mobility may arise as cartilage continues to degenerate, significantly affecting everyday activities and quality of life.

➤ **Prognosis:** The degree and amount of joint deterioration, comorbidities, and therapy interventions are some factors that affect the prognosis of osteoarthritis (OA). Even though there isn't a known treatment for osteoarthritis (OA), symptom management techniques, including physical therapy, lifestyle changes, and painkillers, can help reduce pain and enhance joint function. Surgical procedures, such as joint replacement surgery, could be required in some circumstances to relieve pain and restore mobility in severely damaged joints. Many people with OA are able to effectively manage their symptoms and preserve a high quality of life with the right care.

Rheumatoid arthritis (RA)

➤ **Progression:** Periods of flare-ups (or illness activity) interspersed with remissions are characteristic of how RA progresses. People may have increased joint pain, edema, and stiffness during flares, frequently accompanied by systemic symptoms such as weariness, fever, and weight loss. In the absence of adequate therapy, RA can result in disability, irreparable joint degeneration, and shortened life expectancy.

➤ **Prognosis:** With the development of new treatment methods, such as disease-modifying antirheumatic medications (DMARDs) and biologic therapy, the prognosis for RA patients has greatly improved recently. To maximize results and reduce joint damage, it is imperative that RA be diagnosed early and aggressively managed. Even though RA is a chronic illness, specific treatment plans can help manage symptoms, lower inflammation, and maintain joint function. Nevertheless, some people may continue to develop joint deterioration in spite of treatment, which could result in disability and functional impairment. Rheumatologists and multidisciplinary care teams must closely monitor RA patients to maximize long-term results.

Juvenile idiopathic arthritis (JIA)

➢ **Progression:** The course of juvenile idiopathic arthritis varies according to the particular subtype, severity, and responsiveness to therapy. While some children may have persistent erosive arthritis with considerable joint destruction and functional impairment, others may experience mild, self-limited arthritis that heals with modest intervention. Like adult-onset inflammatory arthritis, JIA can also be characterized by periods of flare-ups and remissions in the illness.

➢ **Prognosis:** A number of factors, such as the disease's subtype, activity, and early therapy commencement, affect the prognosis of juvenile-onset arthritis (JIA). For children with JIA, reducing joint damage and maximizing outcomes require early diagnosis and intensive care. DMARDs, biologic treatments, intra-articular corticosteroid injections, and nonsteroidal anti-inflammatory medications (NSAIDs) are commonly used in conjunction as treatment for joint inflammation (JIA). Many children with JIA can achieve illness remission and have active, productive lives with prompt intervention and comprehensive care. Ongoing monitoring and interdisciplinary care are crucial because some children may endure long-term impairment, joint injury, and persistent disease activity.

Psoriatic arthritis (PsA)

➢ **Progression:** The course of this condition varies significantly among those who are impacted; some have modest joint involvement, while others develop severe, incapacitating arthritis. Numerous joints, including the spine, fingers, toes, and bigger joints like the knees and hips, can be impacted by PsA. PsA can exacerbate the course of the disease by causing enthesitis, or inflammation of tendon attachments, and dactylitis, or swelling of the fingers and toes, in addition to joint symptoms.

➢ **Prognosis:** The severity of the disease, the degree of joint involvement, and the patient's reaction to treatment all affect the prognosis of PsA. Controlling disease activity, avoiding joint damage, and maintaining function depend on early diagnosis and prompt treatment. DMARDs, biologic treatments, targeted therapies, and nonsteroidal anti-inflammatory medications (NSAIDs) are commonly used in PsA treatment regimens. A decent quality of life and symptom control are achievable for many people with PsA with prompt care and management. Nevertheless, even receiving treatment, some patients may continue to develop joint deterioration and impairment, which emphasizes the necessity of regular monitoring and therapeutic adjustments.

➢

Gout Arthritis:

➤ **Progression:** Urate crystal deposition in the joints causes gout arthritis, a form of inflammatory arthritis marked by flare-ups of excruciating pain, swelling, and inflammation. Gout can evolve from sporadic, acute flare-ups to persistent, recurrent bouts of joint inflammation. Gout can cause joint injury, deformity, and tophi (lumps of urate crystals) in the surrounding tissues and joints. It can also develop if left untreated.

➤ **Prognosis:** Several factors, including the frequency and intensity of gout attacks, concomitant conditions, and treatment compliance, influence the likelihood of developing gout arthritis. Dietary adjustments and weight loss are examples of lifestyle changes that can help lower the frequency of gout attacks and avoid consequences. Medications that lower blood urate levels and control acute flare-ups include colchicine, nonsteroidal anti-inflammatory medications (NSAIDs), and urate-lowering therapy. Many gout sufferers can control their symptoms and avoid long-term joint damage and problems with appropriate therapy and lifestyle changes.

Lupus Arthritis:

➤ **Progression:** Lupus arthritis is a result of systemic lupus erythematosus (SLE), an inflammatory disease marked by tissue and organ inflammation. There is sometimes a correlation between the development of lupus arthritis and the overall disease activity of sickle cell disease (SLE), which varies widely across afflicted individuals.

The tiny joints of the hands and feet are usually affected by non-erosive, symmetric polyarthritis when lupus arthritis first manifests. Lupus arthritis may occasionally result in joint deformity, functional impairment, and disability.

- ➢ **Prognosis:** The degree of joint involvement, the activity of the disease, and the responsiveness to treatment are some of the criteria that determine the prognosis of lupus arthritis. The goals of lupus arthritis treatment are to maintain joint function, lower inflammation, and manage the disease's activity. To treat joint pain and stop the condition from getting worse, doctors may use corticosteroids, immunosuppressive medicines, and nonsteroidal anti-inflammatory drugs (NSAIDs).

  Many people with lupus arthritis are able to achieve disease remission and retain a good quality of life with prompt intervention and extensive care. Nevertheless, some individuals may continue to have joint damage and chronic, persistent arthritis even after receiving treatment, necessitating continued observation and therapeutic adjustments.

Fibromyalgia Arthritis

- ➢ **Progression:** Fibromyalgia frequently progresses in an unpredictable manner, with symptoms that change in intensity over time. Fibromyalgia can have a major influence on everyday functioning and quality of life, even while it does not cause joint inflammation or injury.

- ➢ **Prognosis:** The severity of the symptoms, the patient's responsiveness to treatment, and other factors all affect the prognosis of fibromyalgia. A multidisciplinary strategy is commonly employed in the treatment of fibromyalgia, encompassing medicine, physical therapy, cognitive-behavioral therapy, and lifestyle adjustments. Even though fibromyalgia is regarded as a chronic condition, with the right care, many people can experience symptom alleviation and functional improvement.

Continuous support and symptom management techniques are necessary for certain patients, nevertheless, as they may continue to have impairment and symptoms despite therapy. Every type of arthritis presents different characteristics and difficulties, so proactive management, thorough care, and early diagnosis are essential for optimizing long-term results and reducing joint deterioration and impairment.

Recent improvements in treatment methods and ongoing research projects have significantly improved the outlook for many individuals with arthritis. More research is required to fully understand the fundamental causes of arthritis and develop more effective therapies for this debilitating family of diseases.

Chapter 3:
Diet and Nutrition for Arthritis

One of the most asked questions people suffering from arthritis ask is, "Is there a specific arthritis diet?" To address this, there is no special diet that can cure arthritis; some foods can only help lower inflammation, ease joint pain, and relieve other symptoms.

This chapter will address the significance of diet and nutrition in arthritis management. We will examine the effects of food decisions on inflammation, joint health, and overall wellness. Several types of arthritis, such as psoriatic, gout, and rheumatoid, are primarily characterised by inflammation. Though it is the body's normal reaction to an accident or illness, arthritis causes chronic inflammation that, over time, can harm joint tissues.

Dietary decisions are vital in managing arthritis, as some foods can increase or decrease inflammation. No one diet works for everyone when it comes to arthritis, but research indicates that specific eating habits and foods can help reduce symptoms and enhance joint health in general.

It is important to realize that different people with arthritis have different dietary sensitivity and preferences. Although some meals may be beneficial to one individual, they may cause problems in another. Dietary suggestions should be customized to each person's needs, tastes, and medical circumstances. Getting advice from a qualified dietitian or other healthcare professional can assist in creating a customized nutrition plan that effectively manages arthritic symptoms and satisfies specific dietary objectives.

It's important to note that a particular diet can't cure arthritis; dietary changes can only help control symptoms, lessen inflammation, and enhance joint health. A well-balanced, nutrient-rich diet can help people with arthritis feel better and enhance their quality of life. This chapter will guide you through the importance of nutrition and food in managing arthritis.

Foods That Can Have Potential Benefits for Individuals With Arthritis

One of the strategies for managing arthritis symptoms is to be aware of the foods that are beneficial for the condition. Certain food kinds, such as the omega-3 fatty acids found in fish, fruits high in antioxidants, ginger, turmeric, and more, may help reduce inflammation and pain associated with arthritic symptoms.

Certain types of arthritis, like rheumatoid arthritis, may be influenced by dietary considerations. Therefore, modifying your diet may help reduce the symptoms of arthritis.

How Foods Can Help with Arthritis

Arthritis causes a variety of symptoms, including joint swelling, pain, stiffness, and restricted range of motion. For instance, rheumatoid arthritis is caused by an autoimmune malfunction in which the immune system wrongly assaults joint tissues and, in rare cases, other organs. In contrast, osteoarthritis is frequently caused by chronic mechanical load on the joints. This wear and tear eventually erode joint cartilage, causing discomfort and restricted movement.

In certain cases of arthritis, pain, stiffness, and swelling can be significantly reduced by controlling and lowering inflammation. To lessen pain and improve symptoms, medications are frequently used to reduce inflammation linked to arthritis. Some foods are also effective supplementary treatments for arthritis because of their anti-inflammatory qualities.

For those who have rheumatoid arthritis, the Mediterranean diet, in particular, may help ease discomfort and swelling as well as tenderness in the joints. Additionally, researchers in many studies have found that those adhering to a Mediterranean food pattern had a decreased incidence of osteoarthritis pain and symptoms.

Let's take a deeper look at these foods one after the other.

Oily Fish

Oily fish, such as salmon, are known for their ability to relieve arthritic symptoms and enhance joint function. This is partially owing to its abundant omega-3 fatty acids, including EPA and DHA, which have significant anti-inflammatory properties.

Omega-3 fatty acids are essential for regulating the body's inflammatory processes. They help relieve joint pain, swelling, and morning stiffness, typical in arthritis, by decreasing the production of pro-inflammatory cytokines and other inflammatory mediators. Incorporating omega-3 fatty acids into one's diet can assist control of arthritic symptoms and enhance overall health.

Also, oily fish intake has been associated with increased blood flow during exercise. Increased blood flow improves nutrition delivery and oxygenation to the joints, which promotes tissue regeneration and reduces inflammation. This can improve joint function, reduce discomfort, and increase mobility in those with arthritis.

The anti-inflammatory properties of omega-3 fatty acids go beyond joint health. They have been linked to cardiovascular advantages, such as a lower risk of heart disease and stroke, two prevalent comorbidities in people with arthritis. Consuming oily fish can improve the overall well-being and quality of life of people living with arthritis by increasing cardiovascular health.

For those with arthritis, including fatty fish in the diet as part of a balanced and nourishing meal plan can have a major positive impact. Daily consumption can enhance the anti-inflammatory properties of omega-3 fatty acids and promote joint health—ideally, at least two doses each week. It's crucial to remember that oily fish should only be a small portion of a holistic strategy for managing arthritis, including prescription drugs, physical therapy, and lifestyle changes.

Walnuts

Apart from being a tasty snack, walnuts can be an effective ally for managing and reducing arthritic symptoms. Like oily fish, walnuts' anti-inflammatory and high-omega-3 fatty acid content can help reduce arthritis-related joint stiffness and pain.

Arthritis is characterised by joint inflammation, which causes discomfort and restricts movement. Walnuts contain naturally occurring anti-inflammatory compounds known as omega-3 fatty acids, which assist in alleviating joint inflammation and discomfort.

Additionally, eating walnuts can aid in preserving healthy cholesterol levels. High blood cholesterol can worsen the symptoms of arthritis as it is often linked to inflammation. Walnuts indirectly help to reduce inflammation in the body by lowering cholesterol, which aids in the relief of arthritis symptoms.

Walnuts also alleviate hypertension and promote relaxed blood arteries. The improved circulation to the joints and decreased cardiac strain are especially advantageous for those with arthritis, as they increase joint flexibility and function.

A simple and efficient method of controlling arthritic symptoms is to include walnuts in your regular diet. Walnuts provide a quick and delicious way to reduce arthritis-related joint pain and inflammation, whether eaten as a snack or added to salads, oatmeal, or baked goods.

Dark Green Leafy Vegetables

When managing and preventing arthritis, eating a diet rich in dark green leafy vegetables is not only advised but necessary for optimum health. It may come as a surprise, but cruciferous vegetables, such as broccoli and cauliflower, are essential for preventing the development of arthritis and joint pain. Rich in carotenoids, these veggies protect our cells and tissues from oxidative damage by fighting free radicals in the body.

Also, kale, broccoli, spinach, Brussels sprouts, Swiss chard, and Bok choy are green leafy vegetables loaded with essential vitamins like A, C, and K and various antioxidants. In tandem, these nutrients strengthen cells against damage from free radicals, which are known to play a major role in developing inflammation and rheumatoid arthritis. Besides, these veggies' rich supply of calcium keeps bones strong and supports joint resilience and general health.

You can protect yourself from arthritis and other inflammatory illnesses by including dark green leafy vegetables. They are a powerful source of nutrients. By prioritizing these nutrient-rich foods, you can aggressively maintain your joint health and improve general well-being.

Onions and Garlic

Garlic and onions, staples in kitchens everywhere, do more for health than merely add taste to food. They effectively reduce inflammation and ease the symptoms of rheumatoid arthritis, for example. The antioxidant quercetin, known for its anti-inflammatory qualities, is abundant in onions, particularly red onions. Quercetin improves joint health by scavenging free radicals and decreasing inflammation.

Allicin, on the other hand, a substance found in garlic, is known to reduce symptoms of rheumatoid arthritis linked to it. Allicin's anti-inflammatory and immune-modulating properties can relieve joint pain and stiffness. Garlic also includes diallyl disulfide, which is useful for many health issues and may help treat joint-related conditions.

To reduce inflammation and promote joint health, onions provide a tasty, all-natural remedy. These commonplace kitchen items highlight the amazing power of everyday foods to support general health and target particular health issues.

Bone Broth

Nutritional powerhouse bone broth is well known for its ability to support bone density and joint health. Bone broth, high in amino acids containing glucosamine, offers vital components for preserving joint health. For instance, supplementing with glucosamine can help reduce joint discomfort and enhance joint function, especially in those with arthritis. Glucosamine is a naturally occurring chemical that cushions joints.

Calcium is needed for strong bones and osteoporosis prevention; bone broth has enough of it. Regular bone broth consumption promotes bone density and overall skeletal health by ensuring enough calcium intake.

Bone broth is made by heating bones in a gelatinous fluid resembling the natural collagen in tendons, ligaments, joints, and other tissues. By enhancing collagen production, consuming bone broth lowers the risk of injury and enhances joint function by supporting joint integrity.

Regularly consuming bone broth as a supplement or as the foundation for soups and stews can enhance your joints' general health and well-being. Because of its nutrient-rich makeup, it is a beneficial addition to any diet, but it is especially helpful for people who want to keep their bones strong and joints pain-free.

Special Anti-Inflammatory Diet for Arthritis Patients

As previously mentioned, an anti-inflammatory diet is a dietary strategy intended to lessen inflammation, which can be especially advantageous for people with arthritis. An anti-inflammatory diet can support the management of arthritis symptoms by addressing the underlying cause of inflammation and enhancing overall well-being, in addition to medication and other treatments.

The body's natural reaction to damage or infection is inflammation, typified by pain, redness, swelling, and heat. However, inflammation becomes chronic in diseases like arthritis, causing continuous harm to the surrounding tissues and joints.

Because inflammation is a prevalent characteristic of many arthritis conditions, anti-inflammatory strategies are applicable for managing symptoms irrespective of the particular type of arthritis.

The following are the central tenets of an anti-inflammatory diet:

1. Rich with Fruits and Vegetables: An excellent source of antioxidants, vitamins, minerals, and phytochemicals that support cardiovascular health and decrease inflammation are colourful fruits and vegetables. So, go for a wide range of nutrients.

2. Healthy Fats: Consume healthy fat foods like nuts, seeds, olive oil, and fatty seafood (such as salmon, mackerel, and sardines). These fats include omega-3 fatty acids, which have significant anti-inflammatory properties.

3. Lean Proteins: Consume foods like fish, poultry, tofu, and legumes that are low in fat regularly. Limiting or staying away from red and processed meats is best because they can worsen inflammation.

4. Whole Grains: Instead of refined grains and processed carbohydrates, choose whole grains like brown rice, quinoa, oats, and whole wheat. These grains offer fibre and important nutrients.

5. Herbs and Spices: Because of their anti-inflammatory qualities, include herbs and spices like cinnamon, ginger, garlic, and turmeric. In addition to improving food taste, these savoury additions have health advantages.

6. Limit Sugar and Processed Foods: Reduce your consumption of desserts, sugary snacks, processed foods, and beverages with a lot of added sugar. These foods may worsen the symptoms of arthritis and exacerbate inflammation.

7. Hydration: Make sure you stay hydrated by sipping lots of water all day long. Alcohol and sugary drinks should be consumed in moderation as they can exacerbate dehydration and inflammation.

Consider Taking the Following:

- **Omega-3 Fatty Acids:** These are mostly found in fatty fish, including salmon, trout, and mackerel. They are well-known for their anti-inflammatory characteristics. These fats have the ability to lessen inflammation in the body, which may help ease arthritis-related joint pain and stiffness. If you're not a big fish eater, you might want to include some plant-based omega-3 sources, like hemp, chia, flax, and walnut seeds.

- **Turmeric:** Turmeric, a spice derived from the root of the Curcuma longa plant, is well-known for its strong anti-inflammatory properties. Studies have looked at the potential advantages of curcumin, the active component of turmeric, in treating the symptoms of arthritis. To take advantage of turmeric's anti-inflammatory properties, consider including it in food or supplements. Black pepper and turmeric can improve the body's absorption of the latter.

- **Ginger:** Another spice with anti-inflammatory solid qualities, ginger is frequently used to help people with arthritis feel less pain and inflammation. Add fresh ginger to teas, smoothies, or savoury dishes to reap the benefits. For those who would instead take a concentrated form, there are also supplements made of ginger.

- **Berries:** Antioxidants called anthocyanins, abundant in berries like raspberries, blackberries, blueberries, and strawberries, help fight oxidative stress and inflammation. These colourful fruits make a tasty and nourishing addition to an anti-inflammatory diet, whether consumed fresh, frozen or blended into smoothies.

- **Leafy Greens:** This is rich in vitamins, minerals, and phytonutrients that promote general health and lower inflammation; leafy greens include spinach, kale, Swiss chard, and collard greens. Add leafy greens to salads, stir-fries, soups, and smoothies to increase your nutrient intake and support joint health.

- **Cruciferous Vegetables:** Cruciferous vegetables include Brussels sprouts, cabbage, broccoli, cauliflower, and other vegetables that are high in substances that have antioxidant and anti-inflammatory properties. These vegetables are also high in fibre, vitamins, and minerals, which makes them a great complement to a diet that aims to lower inflammation. Add them to your meals by eating them raw, steam-cooked, or roasted.

- **Olive Oil:** This Mediterranean diet staple is well-known for its anti-inflammatory benefits. A common ingredient in the Mediterranean diet is olive oil. Olive oil's high concentration of antioxidants and monounsaturated fats is linked to a reduction in inflammation and protection against chronic illnesses. Olive oil may be used as leading cooking oil or poured over vegetables and salads to improve their flavor and offer additional health benefits.

- **Nuts and Seeds:** Almonds, walnuts, flaxseeds, and chia seeds are nutritional powerhouses, high in antioxidants, heart-healthy fats, protein, and fibre. Some variety of nuts and seeds can help enhance joint health and reduce inflammation. These nutrient-rich additions can be enjoyed as quick snacks or used as delectable toppings to salads, yoghurt, or cereal, providing a delightful and healthy method to improve overall well-being.

- **Green Tea:** Green tea's powerful antioxidant, polyphenol, is a popular beverage that has been demonstrated to lower inflammation and protect against long-term ailments. Regular eating of green tea has been shown to improve general health and reduce symptoms of arthritis. Whether you choose to drink it hot or cold, flavoured or unflavored, green tea ought to be a regular part of your daily routine.

- **Probiotics:** Probiotics are good bacteria that enhance gut health and immunological function and can reduce inflammation. Probiotics can be found in abundance in fermented foods such as yogurt, kefir, sauerkraut, kimchi, and tempeh. These foods can be added to an anti-inflammatory diet to improve digestive health and overall wellbeing.

- **Calcium-rich Foods:** Eat foods high in calcium since they help prevent osteoporosis, a common consequence of arthritis, and preserve strong bones. Consuming calcium-rich foods helps improve bone health and lower your chance of fractures. Some foods include dairy products, plant-based milk enhanced in calcium, leafy greens, tofu, and almonds.

Meal Ideas for an Anti-Inflammatory Diet:

Salmon Salad:

A meal that is high in omega-3 fatty acids and antioxidants can be made by combining salmon that has been grilled or baked with leafy greens, cherry tomatoes, cucumbers, avocado, a drizzle of olive oil combined with a dash of lemon juice. This combination not only adds flavour but also increases nutritional value.

Vegetable Stir-Fry:

To make a dish that is both savoury and anti-inflammatory, sauté a range of colourful vegetables in olive oil with garlic, ginger, and turmeric. Serve this recipe alongside brown rice or quinoa.

Quinoa Salad:

This is a nutritious and energising dish made with cooked quinoa, crisp cucumbers, juicy tomatoes, brilliant red onion, crunchy bell peppers, fresh parsley, and substantial chickpeas. This salad, drizzled with olive oil and lemon juice and topped with feta or goat cheese, is a tasty and nutritious pleasure.

Smoothie bowl:

A colourful and antioxidant-rich smoothie bowl may include spinach, kale, frozen berries, banana, almond milk, Greek yoghurt, and a scoop of protein powder. Top the smoothie bowl with nuts, seeds, and oats for extra crunch and nutrients.

Turmeric-Ginger Soup:

Turmeric-ginger soup is a comforting and anti-inflammatory soup made by boiling onions, garlic, carrots, celery, and turmeric in vegetable broth until the veggies are cooked. It can be served with a side of whole grain bread or crackers. Once the veggies are cooked, the soup is smoothed out with a blender.

An anti-inflammatory diet offers a comprehensive strategy for the treatment of arthritic symptoms by lowering inflammation in the body and enhancing general health and wellbeing. However, people with arthritis should seek the advice of their healthcare experts or a qualified dietitian before making significant alterations to their diet.

Consequently, this guarantees that the diet is based on their health requirements and medical circumstances.

Foods To Avoid or Limit to Manage Arthritis Symptoms

Certain foods should be avoided while adhering to an arthritis diet, as they can worsen joint pain, inflammation, and other discomforts associated with the condition. Foods listed below should be avoided or eaten in moderation:

1. Trans Fats:

These lipids are present in dairy and beef products, albeit in minor amounts. Trans fats, in contrast to High-Density Lipoprotein (HDL), known as the "good" cholesterol, have a negative influence, increasing Low-Density Lipoprotein (LDL), also known as the "bad" cholesterol. The risk of heart disease and inflammation both increased due to height increase. Alterations in HDL and LDL cholesterol levels can also lead to obesity and cardiovascular disease. Your body will have more difficulty fighting arthritis if you consume trans fats. Fried, processed, and fast foods are all sources of these fats. Even though they are only present in trace amounts, it is best to avoid them.

2. Saturated Fats:

Foods containing saturated fats include red meat (beef or lamb), cheese, pepperoni, salami, beef sausages, and butter. Saturated fats are found in other various foods. Saturated fats have the potential to cause inflammation. These fats also increase the risk of developing heart disease. It is recommended that one consumes saturated fats in moderation. They are recommended to constitute less than ten percent of your total calorie intake.

3. Omega-6 Fatty Acid:

In spite of the fact that omega-6 fatty acids are necessary for healthy growth, omega-6 fatty acids are only sound to be sometimes consumed. Avoid consuming an excessive amount of omega-6 fatty acids. Excessive consumption can also cause the release of materials that contain inflammatory properties. Soy, corn, peanuts, nightshades vegetables, fried and snack foods are all sources of omega-6 fatty acid. Minimize the amount of omega-6 fatty acids you consume.

4. Sugary foods:

Refraining from or severely restricting the consumption of sugary foods such as desserts, cold beverages, and pastries may be challenging. However, the effects of sugar are comparable to those of saturated fats. In addition, drinking an excessive amount of sugar raises the risk of developing inflammation. Consuming less sugar leads to a reduction in body weight. The symptoms of rheumatoid arthritis are alleviated when the patient loses weight. It is possible for cytokines, which are proteins that cause inflammation, to be released when excessive processed sugar is consumed.

5. Refined Carbohydrates:

Refined carbohydrates have the potential to promote the production of pro-inflammatory substances within your body. As a result, an inflammatory state is produced. As a result, arthritis is made worse. Bread, cereals, crackers, white rice, white potatoes, and products made from white flour are all examples of foods that contain refined carbohydrates.

6. Gluten:

Individuals who suffer from joint-related diseases experience sensitivity to gluten or casein, which is found in dairy products. Gluten has the potential to trigger an autoimmune reaction in individuals who have celiac disease. Among the foods that contain gluten are rye, wheat, and barley.

7. Alcohol

Drinking too much alcohol can aggravate the symptoms of arthritis and create inflammation, especially in those with gout. Both the effectiveness of medication and the potential for weight gain are negatively impacted by alcohol consumption. When drinking alcohol, it is best to limit your consumption and opt for moderation, selecting beverages with lower alcohol content, such as wine or light beer.

Instead of these foods listed above, you should incorporate whole foods rich in nutrients, lean proteins, healthy fats, and anti-inflammatory foods to support joint health and overall well-being. Individualized guidance and support in developing a diet plan suitable for people with arthritis can be obtained through consultation with a healthcare professional or a registered dietitian.

Healthy Weight for Arthritis Management

Healthy weight is essential for overall wellbeing. It reduces the risk of developing diabetes, cancer, and heart disease. Furthermore, keeping a healthy weight is critical for relieving arthritic pain and improving the efficacy of prescription drugs. Individuals with arthritis can benefit from increased pain alleviation and a better state of health and wellness by prioritising weight management alongside routine medical therapies.

Here are some strategies for achieving and keeping a healthy weight to help relieve your arthritis:

1. Lessen the stress on your joints:

Your joints, especially weight-bearing joints like the spine, hips, and knees, are subjected to increased stress when you carry excess weight. In addition to exacerbating arthritis symptoms, this increased pressure can hasten joint deterioration. You can relieve pain and slow the advancement of joint damage by keeping a healthy weight, which lessens the strain on your joints.

2. Ease Pain: For those who have arthritis, being overweight increases pain and discomfort. The extra pressure on joints may worsen inflammation and improve pain sensitivity. Reduced joint stress from weight loss leads to increased mobility and comfort, which can help ease this pain.

3. Reduce Inflammation: Fat tissue is more than just a passive energy source; it also secretes pro-inflammatory molecules known as cytokines and is metabolically active. The systemic inflammation caused by these cytokines can worsen autoimmune diseases such as lupus, psoriatic arthritis, and rheumatoid arthritis. Weight loss causes the body's fat stores to shrink, which lowers general inflammation levels, lessens arthritis symptoms, and improves disease management.

4. Reduce Disease Activity: Those who are obese tend to have higher disease activity in their arthritis. Gaining too much weight can exacerbate joint damage and inflammation, resulting in more severe

symptoms and a lower standard of living. In order to better control symptoms and increase functioning, losing weight can help lower disease activity and enhance overall arthritis management.

5. Increased Chance of Remission: Studies indicate that obesity and overweight decrease the chance of achieving minimal disease activity or remission in conditions such as psoriatic and rheumatoid arthritis. Reduction of body weight can enhance the efficacy of rheumatoid arthritis medications and raise the likelihood of remission, resulting in better long-term results and enhanced quality of life.

6. Reduced Risk of Gout Attack and Elevated Blood Uric Acid: Gout is a form of arthritis marked by excruciating joint inflammation and elevated blood uric acid levels. There is a significant risk of gout associated with obesity. People with gout can benefit from this condition because it has been shown that reducing body weight lowers serum uric acid levels and decreases the frequency of gout attacks.

7. Slows Cartilage Degeneration in Osteoarthritis:

The degeneration of joint cartilage is the hallmark of osteoarthritis (OA), a degenerative joint disease. Weight gain exacerbates the symptoms of OA and hastens the deterioration of cartilage. You can lessen the severity of your osteoarthritis symptoms and delay the advancement of cartilage degeneration by keeping a healthy weight.

Reducing weight might be challenging if you are overweight, but there are many health advantages to even one activity. In addition to treating arthritis, it also helps to lower the risk of having diabetes, heart disease, sleep apnea, and several cancers. Before you start any weight-loss regimen, make sure you consult your physician.

Chapter 4:
Alternative Therapies for Arthritis

A wide range of non-conventional treatments and activities that provide complementary or alternative approaches to conventional medical care are included in the category of alternative therapies. Arthritis is one of the many health disorders that can be treated with these therapies, which frequently use holistic principles, ancient healing practices, and integrative medical approaches. The primary goals of alternative treatments for arthritis are relief from pain, inflammation reduction, joint function enhancement, and overall well-being. These therapies do not include the use of pharmaceuticals.

Individuals who may receive minimal alleviation or harmful effects from conventional treatments are the target audience for alternative therapies for arthritis. One of the essential purposes of these therapies is to give individuals more options for managing their illness. These therapies emphasise the significance of addressing not only the physical symptoms of a disorder but also the mental and emotional aspects of optimal health, acknowledging the interconnection of the mind, body, and spirit.

Alternative therapies have the potential to mitigate arthritis pain and enhance the quality of life for individuals afflicted with the condition.

Each of these treatments will be discussed in turn in this chapter. There are a variety of non-conventional treatments that have shown success in reducing pain and improving the quality of life for people who are living with arthritis. We will look into the area of alternative therapies for arthritis and provide insights into these diverse approaches. For those seeking supplementary or alternative methods of pain management, alternative treatments offer more options. The management of arthritis necessitates using conventional therapies, including medication and physical therapy.

Notable Alternative Therapies: Acupuncture, Massage Therapy, Chiropractic Care, And Others

1. Acupuncture

This is an ancient practice rooted in Chinese medicine. Due to its medicinal properties, it has become more and more popular today. It entails carefully inserting tiny needles into predetermined body spots to promote energy flow and support the body's inherent healing mechanisms. Acupuncture is especially beneficial for people with arthritis since it can help with pain, inflammation, and tight joints.

Mechanism of action

The release of endorphins, the body's endogenous analgesics, is the mechanism of action that underlies acupuncture's effectiveness in treating arthritis. Through increasing the concentration of these substances, acupuncture helps to reduce arthritic pain. In afflicted areas, the procedure enhances blood circulation and oxygenation, which makes it easier for nutrients to be delivered and toxins to be eliminated. This two-fold effect helps to lower inflammation while also promoting the healing process.

The immune system's reaction to acupuncture contributes yet another level of efficacy in treating arthritis. The technique seems to control the immune system's response, which aids in controlling the inflammatory processes that are a part of arthritis. As a result, acupuncture provides a comprehensive method of reducing the symptoms of many types of arthritis, such as psoriatic, rheumatoid, and osteoarthritis.

Acupuncture's beneficial effects are well-supported by scientific data. It has been demonstrated in several trials to lessen arthritis patients' pain and enhance joint function considerably.

Although acupuncture appears to be a successful adjuvant treatment for arthritis, precautions must be taken. Acupuncture is typically regarded as safe when performed by a trained professional with sterilised needles. There could be mild and transient adverse effects like pain, bruising, or bleeding where the needle was inserted. These side effects, nevertheless, usually go away fast.

Before receiving acupuncture therapy, those with certain medical issues, such as those who have pacemakers, immune system diseases, or blood disorders, should use caution and speak with medical authorities. People can confidently investigate acupuncture as a supplemental treatment for arthritis symptoms as long as they follow safety precautions and acknowledge the abundance of scientific evidence supporting it.

2. Massage therapy

A therapeutic practice known as massage therapy involves manipulating the muscles and soft tissues to release tension, improve circulation, and promote relaxation. It is unique in that it is a commonly accepted alternative treatment for arthritis. It provides relief from the typical joint pain, stiffness, and inflammation.

Mechanism of action

The efficacious mechanism of massage therapy is based on its capacity to elicit diverse physiological reactions. First, manual muscle manipulation helps to relax the muscles, lessening muscular spasms and relieving joint stress and stiffness. For those who are suffering from pain associated with arthritis, this relaxation is essential.

Massage therapy is crucial in improving blood circulation to the afflicted areas. The treatment helps the tissues receive oxygen and nutrients by increasing blood flow, encouraging tissue repair and regeneration. Concurrently, better circulation facilitates the effective elimination of metabolic waste products, improving the general well-being of the tissues in question.

Massage therapy has been linked to psychological advantages and physical benefits. Endorphins and other neurotransmitters may be released due to the process, which would relieve pain and elevate mood. This combined effect on the mental and physical health of arthritic patients emphasises how holistic massage treatment is.

Massage treatment is effective in easing arthritic symptoms. Research indicates that massage treatment can significantly enhance physical performance and reduce discomfort for those with osteoarthritis, rheumatoid arthritis, fibromyalgia, and other kinds of arthritis. One such study was published in the Cochrane Database of Systematic Reviews. As the above review clarifies, its effectiveness in reducing knee osteoarthritis is especially noteworthy.

While massage therapy is a generally safe technique, there are a few things to be aware of. Hiring a certified and experienced massage therapist is essential to guarantee that the proper techniques are applied. For those with specific medical conditions, such as severe osteoporosis, fractures, or deep vein thrombosis, deep tissue massage may need to be avoided. These individuals ought to move cautiously. A healthcare professional should be consulted before beginning a massage treatment regimen for anybody with underlying medical conditions.

3. Chiropractic care

Chiropractic care is a specialist area with a particular focus on musculoskeletal disorders. It has a special position in the medical industry. Chiropractic therapy alleviates pain, enhances general health, and restores proper alignment by manually manipulating the spine and other joints. An increasingly used alternative treatment for the management of arthritis is chiropractic care, particularly for conditions affecting the spine and the joints surrounding it.

Mechanism of action

The primary mechanism behind chiropractic therapy is the correction of misalignments in the spine and other joints, referred to as subluxations in science. These misalignment mistakes may stress nerves, resulting in discomfort and reduced optimal joint function. Chiropractors aim to release this pressure by perfectly applying manual adjustments, improving nerve function and joint mobility. This realignment process is necessary to address the pain, stiffness, and inflammation related to arthritis.

Chiropractors use complementary therapies and spinal adjustments to maximize treatment outcomes. The mainstays of chiropractic care are soft tissue manipulation, therapeutic exercises, and lifestyle counselling. These supplementary treatments support an all-encompassing approach by treating the underlying causes and enhancing long-term musculoskeletal health.

Numerous studies show that, for various arthritic conditions, including osteoarthritis and rheumatoid arthritis, adjustments made by a chiropractor can have noticeable advantages, such as pain alleviation and increased joint function.

4. Physiological Therapeutics.

Safety is essential in any medical procedure, and chiropractic adjustments are no different. Adjustments are usually safe when administered by certified and experienced chiropractors. It is imperative to recognise that severe side effects are uncommon but can include worsening of pain, nerve damage, or herniated discs. Before beginning treatment, a licenced chiropractor must perform a comprehensive examination and assessment to make sure that chiropractic care is appropriate for the patient's needs and condition.

5. Herbal remedies

Herbal treatments have drawn interest because of their ability to reduce arthritic symptoms. Boswellia, ginger, and turmeric are notable among these medicines because of their well-known anti-inflammatory qualities. They provide an all-natural method of easing arthritis-related pain and inflammation.

Mechanism of Action

How herbal treatments work and how well they manage arthritis symptoms are closely related. Curcumin, a potent anti-inflammatory substance, is found in turmeric. Curcumin inhibits several molecular targets involved in the inflammatory process, which may reduce joint pain and inflammation. With a long history of medical use, ginger is a unique spice with anti-inflammatory and antioxidant qualities. Reduced inflammation might result from changes to the immune system. Because they block certain enzymes involved in the inflammatory process, boswellic acids, which are present in the resin of Boswellia trees, have anti-inflammatory qualities. Boswellia receives its name in this way.

These herbal remedies have the potential to help relieve arthritic symptoms, as demonstrated by scientific evidence. Studies on turmeric have shown promise in reducing the symptoms of osteoarthritis and rheumatoid arthritis. However, further research is needed to confirm these findings. Because of its analgesic and anti-inflammatory qualities, ginger may help with pain management and joint function. Preclinical research and clinical trials have shown that Boswellia has anti-inflammatory properties; these findings raise the possibility of using Boswellia in addition to traditional arthritis treatments.

Recognising that some herbs may have negative effects or interact negatively with pharmaceuticals is important, underscoring the significance of receiving individualised advice. For example, supplements containing turmeric with blood-thinning drugs may interact negatively, so use them cautiously. In general, ginger is safe to eat in moderation, but too much of it might cause stomach pain. Although many people tolerate Boswellia well, some may experience stomach problems.

The use of herbal medicines can enhance conventional arthritis therapies. They can provide people with more choices for managing their symptoms. They shouldn't, however, take the place of prescription drugs without first speaking with a doctor. Herbal therapies should be carefully considered with other medications, individual health conditions, and overall treatment goals when incorporated into a complete approach for managing arthritis.

6. Aromatherapy

For those suffering from chronic pain, aromatherapy is a helpful option. Many people report feeling pain relief for several weeks following an aromatherapy massage. These oils, made from plant-based essential oils, can be used topically, ingested, or bathed.

Aromatherapy has several kinds of essential oils, each with a specific purpose. These oils can help reduce inflammation and stop cartilage tissue deterioration, which may be necessary in treating joint discomfort. For instance, an aromatherapy massage with lavender oil may help relieve discomfort for those with osteoarthritis in the knees. Furthermore, ginger, which has long been utilised for its anti-inflammatory qualities, might be a viable substitute for pain relief that is just temporary.

Mechanism of Action

Aromatherapy works by interacting with the body through the use of essential oils. When applied or breathed, these oils cause skin receptors and olfactory system reactions. Compounds included in essential oils may have relaxing, anti-inflammatory, or analgesic properties that help reduce pain.

Even though anecdotal evidence suggests aromatherapy works, scientific research is necessary to comprehend its effects fully. Aromatherapy's potential for pain relief is still being studied. Positive results are suggested by specific research, which highlights the treatment's ability to lessen pain and improve general well-being. More thorough research is necessary to confirm aromatherapy's efficacy, as the current body of evidence is inconclusive.

Prioritising safety above everything else is crucial while examining alternative therapies. While aromatherapy is usually considered safe, there are still certain things to be cautious about. Certain people may experience sensitivities or allergic responses to essential oils because of their high concentration. Before engaging in extended aromatherapy, it is imperative to conduct a patch test and get advice from a licenced aromatherapist or healthcare expert, particularly for those who are pregnant or have underlying medical concerns.

7. Reflexology

Reflexology has gained popularity as a possible substitute for standard opioids in the treatment of arthritis pain. There have been claims that reflexology is just as effective as these medications. This method entails applying pressure to particular body parts, mainly the hands and feet, which are said to represent different bodily functions and systems.

Mechanism of Action

The basic idea of reflexology's mechanism of action is that certain places on the hands and feet, referred to as reflex points, are related to different organs and body components. Practitioners want to encourage equilibrium within the relevant systems and boost energy flow by applying pressure to these reflex spots. Reflexology proponents contend that concentrating on specific reflex points may help lessen pain and discomfort related to joint inflammation in the context of arthritis.

Reflexology is becoming more and more popular as a means of managing arthritis, but before using it, it is essential to evaluate the evidence that is currently available. There are few thorough scientific studies on reflexology and arthritis, and the available ones frequently have methodological and standardisation issues. Although some people experience excellent results and symptom relief from reflexology sessions, scientists still need to be more consensus on reflexology's overall effectiveness.

When assessing the potential of reflexology as an adjunctive method for managing arthritis, safety concerns are crucial. When done by skilled and certified professionals, reflexology is generally considered a safe, non-invasive technique with few adverse effects. Before receiving reflexology treatments, anyone with specific medical concerns, such as circulation problems or foot injuries, should use caution and speak with medical authorities.

Reflexology is a comprehensive practice beyond how it could help with arthritic symptoms. Reflexology's supporters claim that reflexology improves general well-being by encouraging relaxation, lowering stress levels, and strengthening the body's inherent healing abilities. Reflexology may have physiological advantages on arthritis and psychological and emotional symptoms, offering a more complete holistic healthcare approach.

Even though reflexology provides a non-pharmacological option for managing arthritis, people must approach it with reasonable expectations and knowledge of their medical situation. Instead of being considered a stand-alone treatment for arthritis, reflexology should be regarded as an adjunctive approach. A more thorough and customised strategy to treating arthritis symptoms may involve speaking with medical experts, incorporating reflexology into a larger arthritis management plan, and combining medicine, physical therapy, and lifestyle changes.

8. Yoga

Yoga combines diverse postures that improve physical and mental well-being with breathing methods, providing a holistic approach to controlling arthritis symptoms. It has been shown that practicing yoga can help people with arthritis feel less pain and have more strength and flexibility. Yoga combines mindful breathing, gentle movements, and joint awareness to greatly reduce joint stiffness and enhance the overall quality of life for those with arthritis.

The capacity of yoga to lessen joint pain and suffering is one of its main advantages for those with arthritis. To reduce stress and stiffness, many yoga poses concentrate on gently stretching and strengthening the muscles that surround the joints. Furthermore, practicing yoga can help people develop the attentive awareness necessary to manage flare-ups and chronic pain better.

Yoga is essential for building strength and flexibility to preserve joint health and mobility. Regular yoga practice can improve general stability and lower the chance of injury by strengthening the muscles that support the joints. Additionally, the mild stretching exercises in yoga contribute to increased flexibility, which increases joint range of motion and decreases stiffness.

People with arthritis can benefit significantly from specific yoga practices. They concentrate on particular bodily parts impacted by the illness.

For instance, hip-opening poses can increase mobility and lessen hip and pelvis pain. At the same time, mild backbends can help relieve lower back pain, which people with spinal arthritis frequently feel. Similarly, for those who have arthritis in their hands and wrists, poses that target these areas might help reduce discomfort and stiffness.

It's imperative to remember that not every yoga pose is appropriate for people with arthritis, particularly if they have severe joint damage or other medical issues. Yoga must be practiced under the supervision of a trained teacher knowledgeable about arthritis and able to adapt to suit each student's unique needs and limits. Additionally, students with arthritis should be honest with their yoga instructor about any limits or particular concerns they may have in addition to discussing their disease.

Yoga provides psychological and emotional advantages that assist people in managing the difficulties associated with having arthritis. Yoga encourages inner calm, relaxation, and a reduction of stress, which can be very helpful for people managing chronic pain and inflammation. Yoga encourages people to become more self-aware and thoughtful, which enables them to manage their arthritis and enhance their general well-being actively.

Risks And Considerations When Using Alternative Therapies

Alternative therapies can help manage arthritis symptoms, but it's essential to understand that they have pitfalls and considerations of their own. You should be well-informed and cautious when implementing alternative therapies into an arthritis treatment plan. You should consider several aspects to ensure efficacy and safety. The following are some dangers and things to think about when treating arthritis using alternative therapies:

♦ Interactions with Conventional Medications:

Herbal supplements and dietary changes are alternative therapies that may interact with prescription arthritis drugs. For instance, the pharmacological actions of herbal treatments may impair the efficacy of prescription medications or result in unanticipated adverse effects. To prevent potential interactions and guarantee a thorough and safe treatment strategy, healthcare providers must be informed about all treatments, including alternative medicines.

♦ Individual Variability:

Depending on the patient, alternative therapies may or may not be highly beneficial. What is effective for one person might have a different impact on another. Several factors, including the kind and severity of the arthritis, general health, and individual responses to different treatments, influence this heterogeneity. Because of this, people might have to investigate many alternative therapies or combinations to determine which is best for their particular circumstances.

♦ Lack of Standardization:

Standardized protocols, dosage recommendations, and quality control methods need to be improved in many alternative therapies. This may make it difficult to guarantee consistent and trustworthy results. For example, the potency and purity of herbal supplements could differ between brands or batches, producing unpredictable outcomes. This danger can be reduced by using reliable supplement sources and seeking advice from licensed professionals.

♦ Potential for Adverse consequences:

Although many people believe alternative therapies to be natural and safe, some may have unfavorable consequences or trigger allergic reactions. For instance, certain herbal supplements can trigger allergic reactions, create gastrointestinal problems, or have a bad interaction with pharmaceuticals. People must be aware of possible side effects and notify healthcare practitioners immediately if they experience any negative responses.

◆ Delay in Seeking Conventional Treatment:

It might be dangerous to rely only on complementary therapies while postponing or avoiding traditional medical treatments, especially in cases of severe or progressing arthritis. Medications considered conventional, like biologics or disease-modifying anti-rheumatic drugs (DMARDs), are frequently essential for controlling inflammation, averting joint injury, and enhancing overall results. The most successful approach frequently balances evidence-based medical treatments and alternative therapies.

◆ Lack of Regulation and Oversight:

Because some alternative therapies operate in unregulated settings, verifying practitioners' credentials, safety requirements, and moral behavior can be challenging. To reduce the possibility of receiving ineffective or dangerous treatments, people should look for respectable professionals with the necessary certifications, such as qualified massage therapists or registered acupuncturists.

Alternative therapies can significantly contribute to managing arthritis; nevertheless, patients with arthritis must approach these treatments with a critical and knowledgeable perspective. Making well-informed decisions and maximizing their arthritis care can be facilitated by speaking with healthcare providers, remaining current on any hazards, and implementing a comprehensive treatment plan incorporating complementary therapies and evidence-based medicine. Maintain constant contact with medical professionals, be transparent about all treatments being considered, and cooperate to find the safest and most efficient solutions for treating arthritic symptoms.

Chapter 5:
Coping Strategies for Daily Living

No one understands the challenges of arthritis and chronic pain better than those who live with them. The constant pain, joint stiffness, and movement restrictions are the everyday struggles that millions of people with arthritis face. There is hope, nevertheless, considering how dire the situation is. Patients with arthritis can take back control of their lives and work toward better health by developing a thorough understanding of coping mechanisms designed to manage their pain.

In this chapter, we will discuss various coping mechanisms that can help you better manage the challenges posed by arthritis and improve your day-to-day activities. We will examine a thorough plan created to lessen the effects of arthritis on day-to-day functioning. We hope to provide people with the information, abilities, and tools needed to succeed in the face of obstacles connected to arthritis by breaking down these coping mechanisms.

An individual's quality of life, relationships, state of mind, productivity at work, and general quality of life can all be greatly affected by arthritis pain. This problem goes beyond physical concerns. As a result, coping techniques cover a complete approach that considers the condition's complex nature and extends beyond typical pain management procedures. The necessity for a thoughtful strategy that takes into account each person's unique needs, preferences, and circumstances is evident when it comes to managing arthritis. In order to help people choose and modify solutions that speak to their own experiences and goals, this chapter provides a wide range of coping mechanisms.

Tips For Managing Daily Tasks with Arthritis

The special difficulties that come with having arthritis can affect anything from everyday chores to leisure pursuits. Even simple tasks can appear overwhelming due to arthritis's stiffness, discomfort, and decreased movement. You may, however, efficiently manage everyday responsibilities, preserve your freedom, and improve your quality of life with the appropriate strategies and adjustments.

Assistive Devices

If you have arthritis, you can move around your house more efficiently and safely and handle daily tasks with less discomfort if you make certain adjustments and use specific assistive equipment. When you have to perform the same work daily or often, the little adjustments or tools that promote independence become important.

If you have arthritis, you may find these mobility aids, safety advice, and assistive gadgets useful around the house.

Self-Help Tools for Your Home

Hundreds of assistive devices are available online and at hardware and home goods stores. The location and severity of your arthritis will determine which tools are best for you. See an occupational therapist (OT) with experience treating arthritis sufferers if you need assistance reducing your options.

The following are some top recommendations for gadgets and tips around the house:

- Extended-handle tools: These make it easier for you to dust or clean, reach items on high shelves, and pick up items off the floor.

- Lightweight appliances: Your joints may be less stressed by a simpler vacuum or mop to maneuver and carry.

- Touch-activated light switches: Compared to standard knobs and switches, these may be kinder to your hands and fingers. With an adaptor that you can purchase in the electrical section of the lighting store, almost any electric device may be made to operate on a touch-on or touch-off basis.

- Lever handles: These can be used to replace sink and door knobs, allowing you to use your palms instead of your fingers to grip. (If changing doorknobs is out of the question, consider purchasing a turning tool with a handle that makes it easier for you to grab the knob; some even make gripping keys easier.)

- Foam pipe insulation: To hold with less discomfort and effort, wrap this over the handle of almost any tool, including pens, brushes, spoons, and gardening or cooking items. (Alternatively, use cloth or tape to wrap tool handles.) Additionally, tools with wider, larger handles are available.

- Spring-loaded scissors: These can make cutting easier. These can facilitate cutting.

Other resources and advice that could be useful to you in various areas of your house include:

In your kitchen:

- Consider using pots and pans with two handles in the kitchen for easy carrying. Some rocker knives, which can make slicing simpler, have two handles.
- Electric appliances, such as can openers, food processors, blenders, and dishwashers, can conserve energy and reduce hand tension when doing tasks like twisting lids, scrubbing, mixing, and chopping.
- Use a non-skid gripper mat when manually opening jars or mixing foods to prevent slips.
- A bottle brush is helpful in washing mugs and glasses.
- Using a cart with wheels makes transporting heavy goods like dishes and grocery bags easier.

In your bedroom

- Zipper pulls and button hooks can assist you in fastening things.
- Long-handled shoehorns might reduce the need to reach and bend when dressing your feet.

In your restroom

- Use a bath stool to sit instead of standing, which can be tiring or straining on joints.
- Use bath mitts to hold slippery soap.
- Use an electric toothbrush and floss holder for easier teeth cleaning.
- Grab bars promote stability.

Tips to Prevent Slips and Falls

Some types of arthritis, particularly knee or hip osteoarthritis, increase your risk of falling and breaking a bone. These strategies will help you reduce your chances of falling at home.

- Remove throw rugs, especially if you use a walker or cane that can catch on the edges.
- Improve lighting. Ensure rooms and staircases are well-lit, especially at night. Small step lights are available at any home improvement store that offers lighting.
- Adding a handrail to any exterior steps going to your home is also a good idea.
- Think about ladders. Use a firm step stool with a wide base if you need to climb. Ideally, it should include a handle to aid with balance.
- Immediately clean up spills and avoid slick surfaces.
- For better stability, use shoes with non-slip soles and sufficient support. Wearing socks or footwear with slippery bottoms is not recommended, especially on smooth surfaces such as hardwood or tile floors, as they increase the chance of slipping.
- Organize clutter by removing potential tripping hazards such as electrical cords, toys, and furniture. Make sure your furniture is placed in a way that makes it easy to navigate, especially if you require mobility aids like a walker or cane.
- Use grab bars and a shower chair to prevent slips and provide stability. A higher toilet seat can also make it easier to sit and stand, lowering the risk of falling in the lavatory.
- Practice effective balancing exercises: Take up yoga, i-chi, or other workouts that build strength and balance. By lowering

your chance of falling, these exercises can help you stay stable
and respond to abrupt changes in posture or uneven terrain
more skillfully.

- Review medications often: As a side effect, several drugs
  might impair balance or induce dizziness. Discuss any possible
  hazards and go over your prescription regimen with your
  healthcare professional. Changing your medicine or dose may
  help lessen these side effects and lower your chance of
  falling.

Other safety precautions to think about include:

- An adjustable transfer bench is used to assist in getting in and
  out of the bathtub.
- Attach grab bars to the sides of toilets and baths.
- Use an elevated toilet seat if you have trouble sitting or
  standing back up.
- Line the bathtub or shower with non-skid strips or a rubber
  suction pad.
- Clear the floor of any debris.

Mobility Devices and More

If your arthritis makes it difficult to walk, consult a physical therapist
(PT). They can determine if you might benefit from an assistive tool or
technology that allows you to move more freely -- but that's not all.

Physical therapists can assist you with the following:

- Reduce pain.

- Ensure optimal joint function.

- Start a specific exercise program to improve strength, mobility, and function.

- Plan for future requirements.

If your physical therapist believes that a mobility gadget or assistance may benefit you, they may discuss one or more of the following:

Cane

Cane can be particularly useful for relieving tension on an afflicted hip, knee, or foot on one side of the body. You use the cane on the other side of your arthritic joint. Inform your physical therapist if you have a systemic form of arthritis, such as RA, and your hands are impacted. Unloading your weight on a cane may result in a flare in your hand.

Crutches

Crutches are the next step up from the cane. Some people only need one crutch, whilst others require two. When people think about crutches, they frequently see the wooden ones they get from the hospital after breaking a bone. However, there are crutches known as strand crutches, which are actually forearm crutches and do not go below your arms. There is a cuff around your forearm. Then, your hand rests on a handle similar to a cane but with far better stability.

Walker

This two-handed device is the next step up from crutches. Someone who has joint difficulties on both sides of their lower body and struggles with balance may benefit from using a walker. A physical therapist can modify a walker to reduce strain and tension on your shoulders, elbows, hands, and wrists.

There are different types of knee braces available for arthritis. Your physical therapist may recommend one to:

- Align your knee
- Relieve pain
- Assist in recovery from knee surgery
- Provide a sense of comfort and support

Air splint

This compression device prevents your ankle from flexing and rolling. These are commonly worn by people who sprain their ankles, but they are also highly useful if your ankle is flared up with arthritis.

Shoe inserts

These gadgets you slide into your shoes can help relieve foot pain if you have rheumatoid arthritis or lower-body osteoarthritis. They may also help to decrease knee osteoarthritis progression.

Orthopedic shoes

If you begin to develop several foot or toe deformities as a result of arthritis, these customised shoes may be a more supportive option.

Adaptive equipment

Adaptive equipment is a vital lifeline for people living with arthritis. They provide diverse equipment, technologies, and machinery to improve daily life and relieve pain. Adaptive technologies are important in improving independence, comfort, and quality of life for arthritis patients, whether negotiating mobility issues, doing everyday tasks, or engaging in leisure activities.

Adaptive equipment includes any instrument, device, or machine designed to help people with disabilities complete daily chores. Adaptive devices are vital aids for people with short or long-term disability, especially those with arthritis.

Types of Adaptive Equipment that Can Help Your Arthritis Condition:

1. Mobility Equipment: Adaptive equipment improves independence and mobility for arthritis sufferers. This category contains a wide range of gadgets, including wheelchairs and wheelchair-accessible vehicles. Mobility aids help people with arthritis traverse their surroundings safely and comfortably, lowering the risk of falls and injury.

2. Daily Living Aids: These products help people with arthritis accomplish daily chores more efficiently. These include bath railings, reaching devices, hearing aids, feeding assistance, and other adapted devices developed to address the specific needs of arthritis patients. Daily living aids help people with arthritis keep their freedom and dignity by tackling typical obstacles such as dressing, bathing, grooming, eating, and toileting.

Some examples of adaptive equipment for everyday living include dressing sticks, sock aids, long-handled shoe horns, bath chairs or shower stools, handheld showers, grab bars, toilet aids, non-skid bowls, plate guards, and non-slip bowls. Dressing sticks are also known as sock aides.

3. Equipment for Instrumental Activities of Daily Functioning (IADLs): IADLs are activities that go above and beyond the bare minimum to improve everyday functioning. Examples of these activities include safety, communication, enjoyment, and cognition. This category of adaptive devices includes amplified phone equipment to help with communication management, hearing aids, screen readers, communication boards, and speech-generating devices. Adaptive toys and sporting goods provide chances for leisure activities that can be enjoyable and relaxing. Further easing the minds of arthritis sufferers and their careers are safety-focused gadgets like wearable call buttons and fall detection systems.

Adaptive Equipment Is Important for People with Arthritis:

- Enhanced Independence: Using adaptive equipment helps people with arthritis carry out everyday chores independently, fostering a sense of independence and self-assurance.
- Better Quality of Life: Adaptive devices help arthritis sufferers live more comfortably and effectively by reducing their physical difficulties. This enables them to participate more completely in social and everyday activities.
- Reduced Pain and Discomfort: Many adaptive equipment are made expressly to lessen joint and muscle strain, lessening pain and discomfort related to daily activities and arthritis flare-ups.
- Injury Prevention: Mobility assistance and safety-focused gadgets enhance general wellbeing by decreasing the chance of falls and injuries.
- Enhanced Participation: By facilitating leisure activities, preserving social relationships, and pursuing interests and hobbies, adaptive equipment helps people with arthritis improve their mental and emotional health.

A key component of helping people with arthritis manage everyday activities, preserve their independence, and enhance their quality of life is adaptive equipment. Adaptive technologies enable those with arthritis to live a more comfortable, self-assured, and active lifestyle by addressing the particular challenges the condition presents. This helps the users overcome obstacles in life with more resilience and ease.

Techniques For Conserving Energy and Reducing Joint Strain

For people with arthritis to properly manage their symptoms and preserve their quality of life, energy conservation and joint strain reduction are crucial techniques. Patients with arthritis can reduce discomfort, avoid flare-ups, and save their energy for the things that matter by using strategies that reduce strain and stress on their joints.

 These numerous methods and lifestyle adjustments will help you save energy and lessen joint stress.

Pacing Practices: Pacing activities is an important strategy for patients with arthritis. This entails dividing work into manageable chunks and alternating action periods with rest. People can lessen the strain on their joints and avoid fatigue by spreading their energy throughout the day without overexerting themselves.

Joint-favourable Positions: Choosing favourable positions for the joints might hehelpstrain when engaging in activities. For example, it is more equitable to spread the burden while lifting objects using larger joints, such as the knees and hips, rather than the tiny joints in the hands. It's crucial to maintain good body mechanics, and joint-friendly postures can be achieved with the help of adaptable equipment like ergonomic tools or supportive braces.

Assistive equipment: Making use of assistive devices is a crucial tactic for reducing joint stress and energy consumption. Extra support is provided by equipment like wheelchairs, walkers, and canes, which lessens the strain on weight-bearing joints. Tools with ergonomic designs, such as reach extenders or jar openers, can help make daily chores easier and less stressful on arthritic joints.

Energy-Efficient Movement: For individuals with arthritis, understanding and putting into practice energy-efficient movement patterns can greatly improve their quality of life. In order to reduce needless tension on the joints, this entails using softer, more controlled actions. Occupational therapists are qualified to advise on appropriate movement practices based on the needs of each client.

Time management: For arthritis sufferers to balance activity and relaxation times, effective time management is essential. Setting priorities and managing your energy consumption can help you avoid burnout. Maintaining endurance and avoiding overexertion is possible by planning intervals between activities that provide enough recovery.

Adaptive Seating and Sleeping Arrangements: Adaptive sleeping and seating arrangements are essential for minimizing joint strain. Make sure your sleeping and seating arrangements are comfortable. Adequately cushioned and equipped with adjustable features, supportive chairs can enhance posture and reduce pressure on the hips and spine. Furthermore, improving sleep quality and promoting total energy conservation can be achieved by utilizing ergonomic pillows and mattresses customized to each person's comfort preferences.

Temperature Regulation: Patients with arthritis may have joint stiffness and pain in response to excessively high or low temperatures. It can be easier to feel less uncomfortable if the room temperature is steady and comfortable, especially when sleeping. In order to reduce inflammation and comfort joints, ice compresses or warm baths can also be utilized.

Weight Management: Staying below a healthy weight puts additional strain on joints that support body weight. Maintaining a healthy weight and general joint health can be facilitated by following a balanced diet and doing low-impact activities like swimming or mild yoga.

Joint Protection Techniques: Joint strain can be considerably reduced by being aware of and implementing these procedures. This includes utilizing larger joints for activities, avoiding repetitive motions, and integrating joint-friendly products and methods into regular duties. Occupational therapists are qualified to offer individualized advice on joint protection techniques.

Emotional Well-being: For those with arthritis, controlling energy levels requires attending to emotional well-being. Anxiety and stress can make pain and exhaustion worse. Energy conservation is indirectly supported by techniques that promote a happy mental state, such as mindfulness, relaxation exercises, and partaking in enjoyable and relaxing activities.

People with arthritis can live more easily by implementing these energy-saving and joint-strain-relieving measures. Individualized strategies tailored to each person's unique requirements and preferences are crucial. Working with medical specialists, including occupational therapists, can help patients with arthritis feel better overall by offering important direction and assistance in creating energy-saving techniques.

Coping With Emotional Challenges and Mental Health Support for Arthritis Patients

Any type of arthritis or associated disorders can be detrimental to one's mental well-being. The most typical symptoms of this are anxiety or depression. It also functions the other way around. The symptoms of arthritis may intensify due to mental health issues.

People don't always seek mental health care for anxiety because it's frequently thought of as being normal. If anxiety is not managed, it might cause more serious issues. Actually, a person's chance of developing depression may rise if they have persistent anxiety.

Anxiety, depression, and arthritis can all have detrimental impacts on general health and quality of life. Sadness or anxiety can make it difficult for a person to motivate themselves to take adequate care of themselves and go about their everyday lives, let alone manage their arthritis or other medical illnesses. For this reason, individuals with arthritis must manage both their physical and mental health problems.

A holistic approach to managing arthritis must include both obtaining mental health care and coping with emotional difficulties.

Patients with arthritis often face a variety of emotional difficulties, such as:

1. Depression and anxiety: Feelings of melancholy, pessimism, and fear about the future can be exacerbated by chronic pain and movement restrictions.

2. Social Isolation: People who experience physical restrictions may find it difficult to maintain social contact or engage in social activities, resulting in social disengagement and loneliness.

3. Tension and Frustration: Managing arthritis's effects on all facets of life and coping with everyday pain can exacerbate tension and frustration.

Coping Strategies:

1. Open Communication: Sharing emotions and worries with close friends, relatives, or medical professionals can help to validate and support you emotionally. Maintaining open channels of contact can promote a sense of connectedness and lessen feelings of loneliness.

2. Mindfulness and Relaxation Techniques: You can lower stress, encourage relaxation, and enhance your general emotional well-being by engaging in mindfulness meditation, deep breathing exercises, or progressive muscle relaxation.

3. Taking Part in Fun Activities and Hobbies: Taking part in pleasurable activities and hobbies can improve mood, divert attention from pain, and give one a sense of fulfillment and purpose. Creating art, music, or writing are examples of creative outlets that can be used as a means of emotional release and self-expression.

4. Seeking Professional Support: Consulting therapists or counsellors specialising in mental health issues can be a great way to get help with the emotional difficulties of arthritis. Therapy sessions can provide a secure environment for exploring emotions, creating coping mechanisms, and enhancing resilience.

5. Sustaining a Healthy Lifestyle: Making self-care routines a priority, such as consistent exercise, a well-balanced diet, and enough sleep, will enhance general emotional health. Natural mood enhancers called endorphins are released when you exercise, and a balanced diet and enough sleep enhance resilience and stress management.

Mental Health Support:

1. Therapy and Counseling: Consulting with certified mental health specialists for therapy or counseling can offer specific assistance and direction in coping with emotional difficulties associated with arthritis. Cognitive-behavioural methods, mindfulness exercises, and stress reduction approaches could all be used in therapy sessions.

These methods can assist people in acquiring coping mechanisms to manage the psychological strains linked to arthritis, movement restrictions, and the emotional effects of chronic pain. In addition, therapy provides a secure environment for expressing emotions such as grief, worry, or frustration associated with the disease, promoting emotional resilience and improving general wellbeing. Working with a therapist or counsellor can enable people to investigate practical strategies for adjusting to changes in lifestyle, preserving social ties, and developing an optimistic outlook—all of which are critical components of comprehensive arthritis care.

2. Medication Management: To treat the symptoms of anxiety, sadness, or other mental illnesses, a doctor may occasionally prescribe medication. It's imperative to collaborate closely with a healthcare professional to assess the efficacy of drugs and any possible side effects. Following recommended dosages and timings is crucial to maximizing benefits and lowering the possibility of negative responses.

More importantly, keep an eye out for potential drug interactions, especially those with over-the-counter medications and vitamins, as these can affect your general health, balance, and mental clarity. Maintain an extensive record of all the drugs you take, including dosage details, and consult your healthcare physician frequently to discuss any possible difficulties. Notify your doctor right away if you have any strange side effects or health changes while taking medicine so they can conduct additional testing and adjustments. Good medication management is essential for preserving mental and physical well-being and enhancing fall prevention tactics.

3. Teletherapy Services: Those who live in distant places with limited access to mental health resources or who have physical impairments that make it difficult for them to get traditional in-person therapy might benefit greatly from teletherapy services. Teletherapy saves time and energy by removing the need for travel, which increases the likelihood that people with transportation or mobility limitations can attend therapy sessions on a regular basis. Teletherapy also provides a higher level of privacy and anonymity, which can be particularly consoling for people discussing delicate subjects or stigmatized mental health disorders.

The flexibility of scheduling virtual sessions allows people to incorporate therapy into their hectic schedules more efficiently, lowering barriers to receiving help. In general, teletherapy fosters more inclusivity and equity in delivering psychological support by extending access to mental health care.

4. Support Groups: Attending in-person or online arthritis support groups can offer encouragement from people who have gone through similar things as you, as well as peer support and helpful information. Numerous organizations, like the Arthritis Foundation, provide arthritis patients and their caregivers with online forums and information for support groups.

A sense of belonging and community can be provided to those with arthritis through participation in support groups. These support groups give people a forum to talk about their experiences, trade advice on managing symptoms and provide emotional support. People can acquire valuable insights into fall prevention measures customised to their requirements by engaging with peers experiencing comparable issues. Guest speakers, such as medical professionals or physical therapists, frequently address support groups, sharing important information on fall prevention strategies and strengthening and balancing exercises.

Online forums also make it possible for people to communicate continuously and access materials, which guarantees that people can remain informed and connected in between meetings. Active participation in support groups can help people with arthritis improve their ability to manage their condition and lower their risk of falling, all while creating enduring relationships within the arthritis community.

Managing emotional difficulties and getting mental health care are essential parts of managing arthritis holistically. Patients with arthritis can enhance their general emotional well-being, manage stress, and become more resilient with the help of these coping skills. People must prioritize their mental health, get help when they need it, and understand that maintaining emotional stability is crucial to living well with arthritis.

Importance of Social Support Networks and Community Resources for Coping with Arthritis

We all value being surrounded by individuals who understand us, make us feel loved and supported and are ready to lend a helping hand when needed. However, for persons with a chronic disease, such as arthritis, a solid social support system is even more important for their overall well-being and health.

Social assistance can take various forms. It could be as easy as knowing your friends and family care about you and that they have your back. It could be something more tangible, such as when your partner cleans the house so you can relax. Support can also take the shape of information: advice, tips, tactics, and tools to help you live better every day.

The importance of social support:

You need assistance in any form it may take. Experts have demonstrated that persons with chronic conditions with a strong social support network have a higher quality of life than those without. Support helps alleviate stress's psychological and physical effects, whether informal or official.

> ➢ Emotional Well-being: Living with arthritis requires managing physical and emotional symptoms. A strong social support network is essential for expressing feelings and receiving emotional validation. Having friends, family, or a support group who understand and empathise with the daily hardships of arthritis can tremendously impact emotional well-being.

Sharing experiences and concerns in a supportive setting promotes a sense of belonging and alleviates loneliness.

> Stress Reduction: Arthritis can cause persistent stress, exacerbating symptoms and affecting health. Social support functions as a stress reliever by giving individuals coping strategies, encouragement, and a sense of security. A supporting network, whether through companionship, shared hobbies, or simply having someone to talk to, can help reduce stress's detrimental impacts on mental and physical health.

> Practical Assistance: Arthritis can cause physical limits, making regular tasks difficult. A robust social support system can provide practical aid such as help with housework, transportation to medical appointments, and grocery shopping. This physical help not only alleviates the stress on arthritis patients but also improves their capacity to navigate daily life more independently.

> Improved medication Adherence: Family and friend support increases medication adherence for arthritis patients. Having a support network motivates people to stick to their treatment plans, whether taking prescribed medications, going to physical therapy, or changing their lifestyle. This leads to better symptom management and overall health outcomes.

> Social support networks offer opportunities to share knowledge, guidance, and coping strategies. Individuals with arthritis frequently encounter unique problems, and learning from others who have been through similar experiences can be empowering. The exchange of information within a supportive group, whether through personal experiences,

symptom-management techniques, or recommendations for healthcare providers, improves the collective understanding and resilience of arthritis patients.

Community Resources

Along with interpersonal interactions, community resources are crucial in supporting individuals with arthritis. Local support groups, non-profit organisations, and internet forums dedicated to arthritis activism and education are examples of such resources. Community resources provide a broader network of information, services, and advocacy initiatives to supplement the help supplied by personal connections.

- Support Groups:

Arthritis support groups, whether local or online, bring together others dealing with similar issues. These meetings allow individuals to share their experiences, discuss coping strategies and foster community. Support groups provide a safe space to express their frustrations, seek advice, and connect with others who are undergoing the challenges of living with arthritis.

- Community resources

Community resources provide educational programmes and workshops on arthritis management, symptom reduction, and overall well-being. These programmes offer vital information, tools, and resources to help people with arthritis take an active role in their health. Educational activities help to raise awareness, self-efficacy, and informed decision-making.

- Advocacy and Awareness Campaigns:

Arthritis-focused organisations utilise advocacy and awareness campaigns to increase understanding, decrease stigma, and influence policy changes. Community resources actively participate in projects aimed at improving the lives of people living with arthritis, campaigning for research, accessibility, and healthcare policies that benefit the entire arthritis community.

The value of social support networks and community services in coping with arthritis cannot be emphasised. These features help to increase mental well-being, reduce stress, provide practical support, promote treatment adherence, and share helpful information and coping skills.

Chapter 6:
How to Cope with Flares and Disease Progression

Having an arthritis flare can feel like hitting a wall. Your arthritis had been tolerable until abruptly swollen joints, pain, exhaustion, and mental fogginess disrupted your daily routines.

For some people, flares are an unavoidable part of their arthritis journey. They are usually transient, but it can be challenging to understand if this sudden increase in symptoms will pass or if it is a warning that you need to change your treatment strategy to prevent your condition from progressing further. Depending on the circumstances and your medical history, your doctor may conclude that it suggests a worsening of your disease and modify your medication.

How you feel a flare may differ based on the type of arthritis you have and the trigger. Some triggers may be obvious. For example, suppose you overexert yourself while working in the garden, exercising more strenuously than usual, or going through a stressful event like moving or changing jobs. In that case, you may suffer a temporary repeat of symptoms. For some people, consuming certain foods or having their teeth cleaned might cause a flare or brief worsening of symptoms.

In other circumstances, a flare may occur unexpectedly and without apparent cause. This could suggest that your medication is no longer effective and should be changed or stopped.

Imagine you've been feeling great, barely thinking about your chronic pain, and then all of a sudden, an arthritis flare strikes you like a tonne of bricks. These periods of increased disease activity are physically and emotionally taxing, especially since they might occur suddenly. If you have osteoarthritis or an inflammatory type of arthritis, such as rheumatoid arthritis, you will likely understand what we are saying.

So, how do you deal with arthritic flare-ups when they occur? Relax; this chapter contains all the answers to any queries you may have had.

In this chapter, we'll look at the details of arthritis flares and disease development. We will discuss effective flare management and coping strategies and how to navigate the difficulties of living with arthritis. Let's get to it!

Arthritis Flares and Triggers

Arthritis flares can be a difficult chronic condition to manage. You may feel great one day and then experience pain and inflammation the next. These unforeseen events can be frustrating and perplexing. Understanding what causes arthritic flare-ups is of the utmost importance for efficient management of the condition.

What Causes Arthritis Flare Ups?

Arthritis flare-ups can be caused by various reasons, which differ from person to person. Here are a few common causes:

- Emotional and physical stress can trigger inflammation, resulting in a flare-up.
- Infections can activate an immunological response, leading to joint inflammation and pain.
- Some diets have the potential to increase inflammation in the body, which exacerbates the symptoms of arthritis. For

example, processed foods, saturated fats, and high amounts of sugar trigger flare-ups.

- Temperature and humidity changes can cause flare-ups. Some people with arthritis suffer more pain and stiffness in cold weather, while others may feel it in humid and hot environments.
- Prolonged inactivity can weaken muscles around joints, increasing the risk of flare-ups.
- Repetitive movements, particularly in already injured joints, can lead to flare-ups from arthritis.

Certain drugs may exacerbate arthritic symptoms. Corticosteroids, for example, can thin the bone, increasing the risk of fracture and joint injury.

To reduce the frequency of your arthritic flare-ups, you must first identify the factors that produce them. Keeping a journal and noting changes in your symptoms might help you detect patterns and make lifestyle adjustments as needed.

Weather and Arthritis Flare-ups

Weather variations can significantly affect the symptoms of arthritis. Many people with arthritis describe feeling more uncomfortable and stiffer in colder, wet weather, while others report flare-ups in hotter, muggy weather.

Although the precise cause of this is unknown, variations in temperature and barometric pressure may impact joint fluid, leading to pain and discomfort. Furthermore, variations in the weather can affect our immune systems and increase our susceptibility to flare-ups.

In case you experience symptoms of arthritis due to weather, there are some things you may do to manage your condition better:

- Avoid dehydration, as it can worsen the symptoms of arthritis.

- Dress according to the weather, putting on loose, breathable clothing in the summer and layers to stay warm in the winter.

- Apply heat or cold therapy to relieve aching joints, depending on the weather. For instance, in cold weather, a warm bath or heating pad may assist in easing discomfort; in hot weather, a cold compress may be useful.

- Refrain from pushing yourself excessively when the weather is bad. Pay attention to your body and take breaks.

If your symptoms flare up due to the weather, think about talking to your doctor about drugs or other therapies that can help control them.

Keep in mind that each individual with arthritis is different, so what works for one may not work for another. To determine the optimal management strategy for your specific needs, it's imperative to pay attention to your body's signals and collaborate with your physician.

What a Flare Feels Like with Different Arthritis

A. Rheumatoid Arthritis

You may experience some of the same symptoms you experienced when your RA diagnosis was made, such as stiffness and pain in the joints, exhaustion, redness, and mental fogginess in the morning. If the same joint becomes painful again, your doctor might want to detect inflammation markers in your blood or perform joint imaging, such as an MRI or ultrasound.

B. Juvenile Idiopathic Arthritis (JIA)

Depending on the severity and subtype of the disease, flare-ups in juvenile idiopathic arthritis patients can present in many ways. Joint pain, edema, stiffness, weariness, and decreased range of motion are typical signs of a flare. During flare-ups, children and teenagers with JIA may also have systemic symptoms such as fever, rash, and generalized malaise. To minimize long-term joint damage in young children with juvenile-onset arthritis, they must keep an eye on their symptoms and seek medical attention promptly.

C. Fibromyalgia Arthritis

"Fibro fog" refers to the abrupt onset of cognitive difficulties, exhaustion, and widespread discomfort during flare-ups. During flares, people may become more sensitive to touch, temperature changes, and mental stress. During flare-ups, other symptoms, such as headaches, gastrointestinal issues, and sleep disturbances, may also get worse. Medications, modification of lifestyles, and coping mechanisms are frequently used to treat fibromyalgia flare-ups in an effort to reduce symptoms and enhance the general quality of life.

D. Osteoarthritis:

This type of arthritis is not systemic in nature, in contrast to other types. It only affects certain joints, not the body as a whole. Even so, especially after overuse, you may experience an abrupt rise in joint pain or edema. Get in touch with your healthcare practitioner if you experience painful episodes frequently. They may suggest that you see a physical therapist or orthopedist.

E. Psoriatic arthritis:

You can have a rise in psoriatic plaques, discomfort, oedema, and possibly even weariness in one or more joints. Keep an eye out for further symptoms because psoriatic arthritis, like RA, can also harm organs. For instance, you should see an ophthalmologist if you experience blurred vision or eye pain.

F. Ankylosing Spondylitis:

Flares of ankylosing spondylitis can cause pain in various joints, including the hands, feet, shoulders, and hips, in addition to typical symptoms of exhaustion and back pain. Never disregard vision issues or other symptoms that can point to the disease's systemic consequences.

G. Systemic Lupus Erythematosus (SLE):

Symptoms of a flare-up include fever, rash, joint pain, exhaustion, oral or nasal ulcers, tingling or numbness, and headaches. As organ inflammation is a feature of active lupus, it's critical to see your rheumatologist to assess your symptoms and prevent the condition from worsening.

H. Gout Arthritis

A gout flare is often called an "attack" because it causes sudden pain and swelling in a joint — often the big toe. A flare-up may be the initial indication of gout, brought on by an accumulation of uric acid in the body. Take your gout medication if you have been prescribed it. If not, call your doctor and use ibuprofen or naproxen (aspirin might elevate uric acid levels). Drink lots of water, ice the sore joints, stay away from alcoholic and sugary drinks, and steer clear of purine-rich meals like red meat and some seafood.

I. Spondyloarthritis

Fare-ups in this condition can cause decreased mobility, stiffness, and greater back pain, especially in the lower back and pelvis. In addition to enthesitis, which is inflammation of the tendon and ligament attachments, uveitis, which is inflammation of the eye, and skin manifestations like psoriasis, people with spondyloarthritis may also have these symptoms. Spondyloarthritis flares can be brought on by physical trauma, stress, or infections, among other things. In addition to physical therapy and lifestyle changes to enhance joint function and mobility, treatment for flare-ups of spondyloarthritis usually entails medication to control inflammation and symptoms.

Strategies For Preventing and Managing Arthritis Flares

1. Prepare ahead of time

Monitoring flare-ups of arthritis is crucial to figuring out what causes them and putting preventative measures in place. Patients with osteoarthritis (OA) can make proactive preparations by taking some medications during predicted changes, for example, by learning how the weather impacts flare-ups. To preserve disease management, people with rheumatoid arthritis (RA) should place a high priority on adhering to their drug regimen. Furthermore, keeping an eye on eating habits can assist in identifying possible triggers, enabling modifications to reduce the frequency and intensity of flare-ups.

Keeping a symptom journal can help you keep track of flare-ups by recording things like your activity level, food, stress level, weather, and medication compliance. This data makes implementing proactive management measures easier and offers insights into unique flare patterns. People can lessen the effect of flare-ups on their everyday lives and general well-being by foreseeing triggers and adopting preventative action.

2. Take some rest

Rest is essential for controlling arthritis flare-ups because it helps the body heal and reduce inflammation. Prioritizing rest during flare-ups is crucial to halting the worsening of symptoms and accelerating healing. Wearing gloves made for arthritis sufferers and napping are two examples of activities that might help reduce pain and weariness, allowing people to preserve energy and speed up healing.

Relaxation methods that can be incorporated into daily routines, including mindfulness meditation or deep breathing exercises, can help manage flare-ups by lowering stress and encouraging sound sleep. During flare-ups, it's critical for people to pay attention to their bodies and emphasize getting enough rest, even if it means temporarily reducing their obligations or activities.

3. Support Group

Arthritis patients can benefit greatly from the community support and resources offered by organisations like Versus Arthritis (https://www.versusarthritis.org) and Arthritis Action UK (https://www.arthritisaction.org.uk). These sites provide a plethora of knowledge regarding flare-up management and prevention tactics for arthritis.

They also help people connect with others going through similar things, creating a safe space to talk about their experiences, get advice, and find support. Through active participation in these support groups, you can learn useful coping strategies, get access to educational resources, and get emotional support—all of which help you manage and prevent flare-ups of your arthritis.

4. Lessen stress

Stress can greatly worsen symptoms and cause flare-ups; stress management is essential to managing and preventing arthritis. Reducing the impact of arthritis on day-to-day living and preserving mental well-being can be achieved by learning to identify and manage stressors.

Relaxation exercises, guided visualization, and fun hobbies are stress-reduction strategies that can help reduce tension and foster calmness. In addition, asking friends, relatives, or support groups for social support can offer consolation and useful help when things are hard.

5. Use with heat and cold therapy

During flare-ups, temperature therapies, such as heat or cold, can help reduce inflammation and pain from arthritis. Warm baths, heating pads, and heated blankets are examples of heat therapy that can help ease stiffness, promote circulation, and relax muscles. Cold therapy can also numb the affected area, reduce swelling, and relieve pain.

By experimenting with various approaches, you can determine which temperature modality best relieves your particular symptoms. Temperature therapy can be a beneficial supplement to medicine and other management techniques when incorporated into regular self-care practices.

6. Take a break

Mental coping mechanisms are important for controlling arthritic flare-ups because they divert focus from suffering. Taking part in enjoyable and relaxing activities might help divert attention from flare-up symptoms and enhance general wellbeing.

Engaging in hobbies, reading, watching movies, or listening to music during flare-ups can generate a positive focus and be a welcome distraction. People can develop a sense of serenity and resilience in the face of misfortune by practicing mindfulness techniques, such as being present in the moment or pursuing creative endeavors.

7. Mild exercise

While rest is essential during an arthritic flare-up, incorporating a small amount of exercise into everyday activities might help lessen symptoms and improve joint flexibility and mobility. Low-impact activities that can improve circulation, tone muscles, and reduce inflammation without exacerbating joint issues or discomfort include swimming, cycling, and walking.

See a healthcare provider before beginning any fitness programme to be sure it is safe and appropriate for you, taking into consideration your needs and limitations. Among the methods for preventing arthritic flare-ups, physical and occupational therapy are particularly effective since they offer customised plans to target certain problems. These therapy treatments not only provide significant insights but also direction on how to create activity schedules that are both safe and effective.

8. Consult your physician

It's advisable to keep lines of communication open with medical professionals during arthritis flares to address any concerns or changes in symptoms quickly. While self-management techniques can help with minor flares, medical intervention may be necessary for severe or protracted flares to minimize problems and improve results.

Get in touch with a doctor for advice and evaluation if symptoms intensify or continue. Medical professionals can evaluate the intensity of flares, modify medication regimens as necessary, and offer necessary advice on symptom control and flare avoidance. For those with arthritis, early intervention during flare-ups can prevent joint damage, lessen disability, and enhance overall quality of life.

CONCLUSION

Living with arthritis is different from person to person, and symptoms can vary on a daily basis. Treatment and management options also differ depending on the kind of arthritis, its severity, and the areas of the body affected. This diversity emphasizes arthritis's complexity as a group of joint-related illnesses, each with its features, causes, and symptoms. While people's experiences with arthritis vary greatly, one common thread unites them: the absence of a definitive cure.

Arthritis is still a chronic ailment for which there is no known cure, despite tremendous advances in medical research and treatment approaches. For people dealing with the mental and physical effects of arthritis, this fact can be depressing. It also emphasises the significance of treating the illness with a proactive, all-encompassing strategy that prioritises symptom control, functional optimisation, and overall wellbeing.

Arthritis management is best achieved through a multimodal strategy that includes medicinal interventions, lifestyle changes, self-care practices, and psychological support. Treatment options may differ depending on the kind of arthritis, its severity, and the specific joints involved. Rheumatoid arthritis (RA), for example, often necessitates aggressive pharmacological treatments to reduce inflammation and prevent joint damage, whereas osteoarthritis (OA) may benefit from a mix of drugs, exercise, and joint protection strategies.

Medications serve an important role in controlling arthritic symptoms and delaying disease progression. These drugs are intended to relieve pain, reduce inflammation, maintain joint function, and improve overall quality of life. However, they are not without risks and side effects, emphasising the significance of constant monitoring and discussion with healthcare experts to guarantee the best treatment outcomes.

In addition to pharmacological therapy, lifestyle changes are essential in arthritis management. Adapting to individual talents and interests, physical activity is important for preserving joint flexibility, muscle strength, and cardiovascular health. Low-impact workouts like walking, swimming, and tai chi can aid pain relief, mobility, and overall well-being—individuals with arthritis need to keep a healthy weight because excess weight can worsen joint strain and inflammation. A well-balanced diet rich in lean proteins, carbohydrates, and a variety of fruits and vegetables is essential for lowering inflammation and improving joint health. People with arthritis can take preventative measures to lessen pain and improve their overall health by following these nutritional guidelines.

Also, self-care techniques like heat and cold therapy, joint protection, and stress management give people the power to manage their symptoms and improve their quality of life. Simple tactics that can greatly impact day-to-day functioning and symptom control include pacing activities, using assistive devices, and practicing relaxation techniques.

Beyond medical and lifestyle interventions, psychosocial support is essential for addressing the emotional and social aspects of living with arthritis. The mental and overall well-being can be negatively impacted by managing chronic pain, functional limitations, and future uncertainty. Those coping with the difficulties of arthritis may find emotional validation, useful advice, and a feeling of community by reaching out to support groups, mental health specialists, family members, and healthcare providers.

The well-known fact regarding arthritis is that there is no known cure; nevertheless, many ways can be employed to assist patients in managing their symptoms, optimising their functional abilities, and improving their overall quality of life. With this book, you may gain complete control over your health and well-being. This book provides various techniques that can significantly assist you in living full and meaningful lives despite the limitations given by this chronic condition.